PELVIC FLOOR

EXERCISES FOR WOMEN

A Step-by-Step Illustrated Workouts to Enhance Core Stability, Reduce Pain, and Improve Bladder Control

Haley S. Ruell

Copyright © Haley S. Ruell, 2024

Disclaimer

The information provided in this book is for general informational purposes only. The author and publisher make no representations or warranties regarding the accuracy or completeness of the information provided herein. The author and publisher will not be liable for any errors or omissions in this information nor for the availability of this information. The author and publisher will not be liable for any losses, injuries, or damages from the display or use of this information.

This book is not intended as a substitute for professional advice. Readers should consult with a qualified professional for advice concerning specific situations. The author and publisher disclaim any and all liability for any reliance on the information provided in this book.

TABLE OF CONTENTS

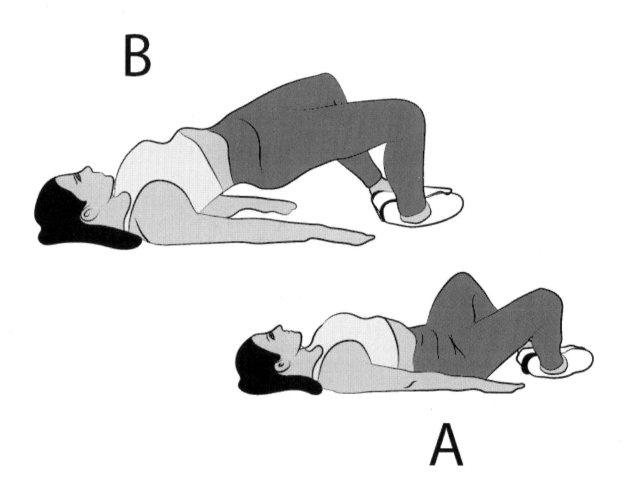

INTRODUCTION

My years of experience as a teacher of women's health and fitness have afforded me the chance to collaborate with a vast number of women at every stage of their lives. My own personal experience has shown me that the health of the pelvic floor may enhance not only one's physical health but also one's mental and emotional well-being. The beginning of my journey with pelvic floor exercises occurred a long time before I became aware of how significant they ultimately were.

During the beginning stages of my professional career, I worked with patients who suffered from a wide range of pelvic health disorders. These diseases included urine incontinence, pelvic pain, trouble recovering after childbirth, and menopausal symptoms. The symptoms that these women experienced often left them feeling unhappy, alone, and embarrassed. I saw a consistent trend. They were nevertheless coping with an illness that had a substantial influence on their quality of life, despite the fact that they were committed to maintaining a healthy lifestyle and engaging in physical activity. I was aware that I wanted to enquire more about the pelvic floor and the ways in which it influences overall wellbeing.

After making the decision to seek specialized training in pelvic floor therapy and exercise, my career growth took a significant turn for the better. I discovered not only about the construction and function of the pelvic floor, but also how it is related to our core strength, posture, and even our mental well-being. The more I understood, the more I began including pelvic floor exercises into my clients' regimens. An increase in self-assurance, an improvement in body awareness, relief from chronic pain, and, most importantly, a reclaiming of their own bodies were the astounding results that were achieved.

My decision to write this book was significantly impacted by the support of a certain customer in particular. She to me postpartum, feeling dismayed by the changes in her body. We began a careful, sensitive process of regaining her strength from the inside out, beginning with her pelvic floor. Week after week, I witnessed her get stronger, not just physically but also emotionally. She highlighted how the exercises had helped her reclaim control not only of her bladder, but also of her life. This episode, among many others, strengthened my devotion to empowering women via pelvic floor health.

This journey has also involved my own physical body. Like many women, I've experienced times when I felt distanced from my pelvic health, whether due to stress, lifestyle changes, or age. By completing these exercises and putting them into my normal routine, I experienced a sense of balance and inner strength that I had never felt before.

This book represents the apex of what I've learned and taught over the years. It's more than merely a set of exercises; it's a guide to understanding and restoring your pelvic health. My objective is to empower you with the knowledge, skills, and support you need to succeed on your journey. Whether you are postpartum, nearing menopause, or simply want to enhance your body, this book will help you connect with your pelvic floor, develop strength, and gain confidence in your everyday life.

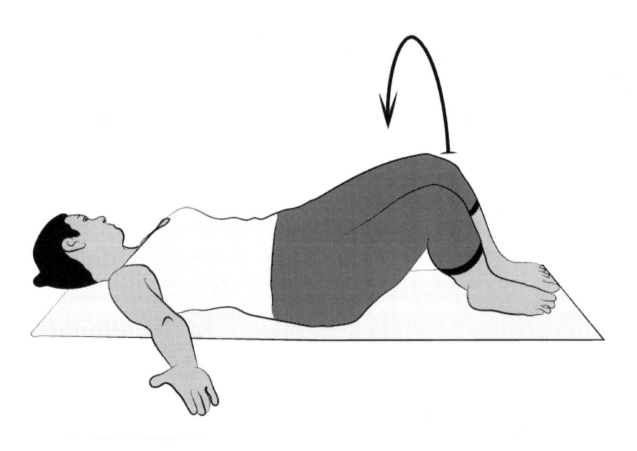

CHAPTER ONE

The Pelvic Floor: Anatomy and Function

The rectum, bladder, and uterus are supported by the pelvic floor, a complex network of muscles, ligaments, and connective tissues that covers the base of the pelvis. Women's basic structural integrity, sexual function, and control over their bowels and urine depend on these muscles. The first step to improving the strength and effectiveness of the pelvic floor is to comprehend its anatomy.

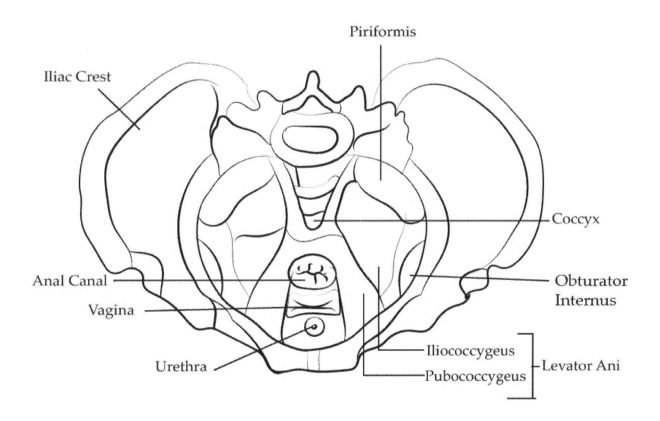

1. Pelvic Floor Muscle Layers

The superficial perineal and deep pelvic diaphragm are the two layers of the female pelvic floor muscles.

The muscles that surround the urethra, vagina, and anus openings comprise the superficial perineal layer. This stratum's main muscles are:

- Bulbocavernosus (Bulbospongiosus): This muscle controls arousal and sexual function and surrounds the vaginal opening. Additionally, it helps with urethral closure, which facilitates urine management.
- Ischiocavernosus: This muscle helps sustain the clitoral erection during sexual stimulation and runs along the pubic bone.
- The external genitalia are supported and the pelvic floor is stabilized by the superficial transverse perineal muscles, which extend across the pelvic outlet.

The muscles that make up the deep pelvic diaphragm form a broad, supportive hammock over the pelvis. This stratum's main muscles are:

- **Levator Ani:** The pubococcygeus, puborectalis, and iliococcygeus muscles comprise the pelvic floor. Together, these muscles maintain continence, support the pelvic organs, and aid in delivery.
- **The pubococcygeus** muscle, which encircles the urethra and vaginal walls, is essential for bladder control.
- **Puborectalis:** It helps with bowel movements and continence by forming a sling around the rectum.
- **The iliococcygeus** muscle preserves the overall structure of the pelvic floor and raises the pelvic organs.
- **Coccygeus (Ischiococcygeus):** This muscle stabilizes the pelvis and supports the pelvic organs by joining the coccyx, or tailbone, to the pelvic wall.

2. The Pelvic Floor Muscles' Essential Roles

Together, the pelvic floor muscles perform a number of vital functions, such as:

Maintaining Continence: You may control the release of gas, feces, and urine by using the pelvic floor muscles to wrap the urethral and anus openings. These muscles close the openings and stop leaks as they contract. They loosen up, enabling the bowels and bladder to pass.

Supporting Sexual Function: The pelvic floor muscles of women are crucial for arousal and pleasure during sexual activity. They protect the clitoris during excitation, boost blood flow to the vaginal area, and contract rhythmically during orgasm. Sexual pleasure and sensation may be improved by having strong, flexible pelvic floor muscles.

Stabilizing the Core: The diaphragm, abdominal, and back muscles are all part of the core muscular group, which is based on the pelvic floor muscles. Together, they support the pelvis and spine, reducing the likelihood of lower back pain and assisting in maintaining proper posture.

3. The Interaction of These Muscles

Together with other core muscles, the pelvic floor muscles regulate the pressure within the abdominal cavity. The pelvic floor automatically contracts to offset the increase in intra-abdominal pressure when you cough, sneeze, or lift a heavy object. This movement gives the pelvic organs more support and stops uncontrollable fecal or urine leakage.

The pelvic floor muscles must contract and expand during exercise, delivery, and sexual activity in order to maintain control and allow for mobility. Therefore, it is crucial for overall pelvic health to maintain both strength and flexibility in these muscles.

The Pelvic Floor's Impact on Women's Health

The pelvic floor is vital to women's overall health and well-being. These muscles constitute the foundation of the core and support the bladder, uterus, and rectum, having a major impact on many areas of a woman's life. A strong, healthy pelvic floor improves urinary and bowel control, sexual health, core stability, and overall physical and mental well-being. Let's look at the special roles that the pelvic floor plays in women's health.

1. Supporting the Pelvic Organs

The pelvic floor muscles operate as a supporting sling, holding the pelvic organs (bladder, uterus, and rectum) in their respective locations. This support is vital for protecting the structural integrity of the pelvic region. When these muscles weaken or become dysfunctional, it may result in conditions such as pelvic organ prolapse, in which one or more pelvic organs slip from their natural position, generating discomfort, pressure, and other health concerns. Women may maintain appropriate pelvic organ support throughout their lifetimes by ensuring that these muscles are both strong and flexible.

2. Maintaining Bladder Control.

One of the most well-known functions of the pelvic floor is bladder control. The pelvic floor muscles encircle the urethra, the tube that transfers urine from the body. When the muscles are strong and performing efficiently, they keep the urethra tight to minimize pee leaks, especially during activities that produce abdominal pressure, such as coughing, sneezing, laughing, or exercising. Weak or overstretched pelvic floor muscles may induce stress urine incontinence, which is when pee escapes during specific activities. Frequent pelvic floor workouts aid to strengthen these muscles, enhance bladder control, and lessen the likelihood of incontinence.

3. Supporting Bowel Function.

The pelvic floor muscles are required for both bowel function and bladder control. They restrict stool transit by enclosing the rectum and anus. When the pelvic floor muscles are in great functioning health, they may contract to prevent unpleasant bowel movements and relax to facilitate regular stool evacuation. Fecal incontinence (uncontrolled bowel movements) and constipation may both be caused by muscle dysfunction. Strengthening and learning to coordinate the pelvic floor may help manage these disorders and enhance bowel health.

4. Improving sexual health and function.

The pelvic floor muscles play a key part in sexual function. They surround the vagina and play a significant role in arousal, pleasure, and orgasm. A strong, flexible pelvic floor may promote sexual pleasure by improving blood flow to the vaginal area while also strengthening muscle tone and control. Conversely, tight or weak pelvic floor muscles may produce discomfort or pain during intercourse, reduced sensation, and difficulty obtaining orgasm. Pelvic floor exercises may help with muscle awareness, relaxation, and control, resulting in greater sexual health and enjoyment.

5. Promoting Pregnancy and Postpartum Recovery

During pregnancy, the pelvic floor serves to support and bear the increased weight of the developing uterus. A solid pelvic floor may aid with pregnancy-related discomforts including lower back pain and pelvic pressure. During labor and delivery, the pelvic floor muscles expand to assist the baby to enter the birth canal. These muscles may become weaker or stretched after delivery, leading in issues such as urine incontinence or pelvic organ prolapse. Pelvic floor exercises before and during pregnancy may help retain muscle tone, facilitate a smoother recovery, and minimize the chance of long-term difficulties.

6. Affecting core stability and posture.

The pelvic floor is a vital element of the body's core, acting with the diaphragm, abdominal muscles, and lower back muscles. It assists in the control of intra-abdominal pressure, spine stabilisation, and good posture maintenance. A strong pelvic floor contributes to overall core strength, which is necessary for balance, stability, and daily actions ranging from lifting and bending to preserving an upright posture while sitting or standing. Conversely, a weak or dysfunctional pelvic floor may produce poor posture, back pain, and an increased risk of injury.

7. Promoting Emotional and Mental Wellbeing

Pelvic floor health has a considerable effect on emotional and psychological well-being. Conditions such as urinary incontinence, pelvic pain, and sexual dysfunction may induce humiliation, concern, and a loss of self-esteem. These fears may also restrict a woman's ability to engage in social activities, exercise, or personal relationships, resulting to mental pain and a lower quality of life. Women who learn to strengthen and maintain their pelvic floor muscles may recover confidence, build a sense of control over their bodies, and boost their overall health.

8. Managing Menopause Changes

As women approach menopause, hormonal changes may affect the flexibility and strength of their pelvic floor muscles. A reduction in estrogen levels may induce weakening of the vaginal and urethral tissues, enhancing the chance of pelvic floor dysfunctions like incontinence and prolapse. Practicing pelvic floor exercises at this phase of life may help counterbalance these changes, maintain muscle tone, and promote urinary and sexual health, making the transition simpler.

Common Pelvic Floor Disorders in Women

Millions of women worldwide suffer from pelvic floor illnesses, which may have a considerable effect on their quality of life. These illnesses are generally caused by weaker, hyperactive, or damaged pelvic floor muscles and connective tissues. Because the pelvic floor supports the bladder, uterus, and rectum and is important in bladder and bowel control as well as sexual function, any failure in this area may result in a variety of symptoms and consequences. The following is a thorough look at some of the most frequent pelvic floor disorders affecting women, including symptoms, causes, and potential remedies.

1. Pelvic Organ Prolapse (POP): Overview

Pelvic Organ Prolapse (POP) occurs when the pelvic floor muscles and supporting tissues fail, leading one or more pelvic organs (bladder, uterus, rectum, or colon) to shift out of their regular locations and press against the vaginal walls. This prolapse may create a sense of pressure, heaviness, or even a palpable protrusion in the vagina.

Types of Prolapse

Cystocele (Bladder Prolapse): The bladder protrudes into the front wall of the vagina.

Rectocele (Rectal Prolapse) happens when the rectum bulges into the vagina's back wall.

Uterine prolapse happens when the uterus descends into the vagina.

Enterocele (Bowel Prolapse): The small bowel pushes into the upper region of the vagina.

Symptoms

- Feeling full or weighted in the pelvis.
- A visible bulge or bump in the vaginal opening.
- Urinary incontinence or difficult urinating
- Bowel movement issues, such as constipation or difficulty passing feces. Low back pain
- Discomfort or discomfort during intercourse.

Causes

- Vaginal births may strain and weaken the pelvic floor muscles.

- Menopause: Lower levels of estrogen weaken pelvic muscle suppleness and support.
- Chronic coughing and heavy lifting could produce undue strain on the pelvic floor.
- Genetic factors: A family history of prolapse may raise susceptibility.
- Obesity: Excess weight elevates intraabdominal pressure, weakening the pelvic floor over time.

2. Urinary Incontinence: Overview

Urinary incontinence is the involuntary leaking of urine. It's one of the most frequent pelvic floor issues, and symptoms may vary from tiny leaks when sneezing or laughing to a strong, urgent desire to urinate that is difficult to control. Incontinence may have a considerable effect on one's regular life, including social embarrassment, activity constraints, and mental pain.

Types of Incontinence:

- **Stress incontinence** is the leaking of urine produced by physical pressure on the bladder, such as coughing, sneezing, exercising, or lifting.
- **Urge Incontinence (Overactive Bladder):** A sudden and intense desire to urinate, followed by involuntary urine loss.
- **Mixed incontinence** is the combination of stress and urge incontinence.
- **Overflow Incontinence:** The bladder does not drain sufficiently, resulting in dribbling of urine.

Symptoms

- Leakage of urine during intense activities
- A sudden, strong desire to urinate
- Frequent trips to the bathroom, often without notice
- Bedwetting or Nighttime Urination Causes
- Weak or damaged pelvic floor muscles.
- Hormonal variations during menopause.
- Pregnancy and Childbirth
- Specific medications or medical problems (e.g., diabetes, obesity)
- Bladder or urinary tract infection.

3. Fecal Incontinence Overview.

Fecal incontinence is the inability to control bowel movements, which causes accidental stool leakage. It may range from slight leakage while passing gas to absolute loss of bowel control. This illness may cause physical and emotional discomfort and is commonly connected with pelvic floor dysfunction.

Symptoms

- Unable to control the release of feces or gas.
- Leakage of stool with physical exercise or effort
- Frequent and urgent bowel movements.
- A sense of incomplete bowel evacuation

Causes

- **Childbirth:** Particularly traumatic births can involve tears or injury to the anal sphincter and pelvic floor muscles.
- **Nerve Damage:** Conditions such as diabetes, multiple sclerosis, or spinal trauma might damage the nerves regulating bowel motions.
- **Muscle Damage:** Injury to the pelvic floor muscles from procedures or persistent constipation may impede bowel control.

4. Pelvic Pain

Pain in the pelvic region that is persistent and lasts six months or longer is referred to as chronic pelvic pain. It may be caused to several circumstances, including muscular spasms, nerve irritation, and inflammation in the pelvic floor muscles and organs. Pelvic discomfort may significantly compromise everyday functioning, emotional well-being, and sexual health.

Symptoms

- A continuous or intermittent aching or throbbing discomfort in the pelvic area
- Pain during urination or bowel motions
- Discomfort or discomfort during sexual intercourse
- Stiffness or spasms in the pelvic area
- Sensations of pressure or fullness in the pelvic

Causes

- **Pelvic Floor Dysfunction:** Overactivity or stiffness in the pelvic floor muscles may produce discomfort, tension, and spasms.

- **Endometriosis:** A condition where tissue identical to the uterine lining develops outside the uterus, producing irritation and discomfort.
- **Interstitial Cystitis:** A chronic bladder ailment resulting in pelvic discomfort and frequent, painful urination.
- **Pelvic Inflammatory Disease (PID):** An infection of the female reproductive organs, typically causing persistent pelvic discomfort.
- **Childbirth Injuries:** Tearing or muscle injury after vaginal birth might contribute to long-term pelvic pain.

5. Overactive Pelvic Floor Muscles (Hypertonic Pelvic Floor Dysfunction)

Unlike pelvic floor weakness, hypertonic pelvic floor dysfunction includes extremely tense or constricted pelvic floor muscles that cannot relax adequately. This illness may lead to a number of symptoms, including discomfort, urine and bowel issues, and sexual dysfunction.

Symptoms

- Difficulty beginning urination or sensing incomplete bladder emptying
- Urge to urinate frequently or on a regular basis
- Pain with bowel motions or constipation
- Pain during intercourse or tampon insertion
- Chronic pelvic discomfort, particularly around the perineum, lower back, and hips

Causes

- **Chronic Stress:** Increased stress levels might lead to involuntary pelvic muscular tightness.
- **Repeated Strain:** High-impact activities or repeated muscular usage without proper relaxation might lead to hypertonicity.
- **Physical Trauma:** Injuries, surgeries, or births may contribute to scar tissue production and muscular stiffness.
- **Improper Exercise Techniques:** Performing pelvic floor exercises improperly or excessively without concentrating on relaxation might lead to muscular hyper activation.

CHAPTER TWO

Preparing for Pelvic Floor Exercises

Locate the Muscles That Make Up Your Pelvic Floor

Prior to commencing exercises that target the pelvic floor, it is necessary to first recognize and grasp the muscles that will be the focus of your efforts. A structure that resembles a hammock is formed by the muscles of the pelvic floor. This structure extends across the bottom of the pelvis and provides support for the rectum, uterus, and bladder. Because so many women fail to recognize these muscles, it may be challenging to identify them and stimulate them in the optimal manner. In this section, we will discuss some fundamental but efficient methods for locating the muscles that make up your pelvic floor, which will allow you to make the most of your workout routine.

One of the Most Important Things to Know About Your Pelvic Floor Muscles

Properly locating and activating your pelvic floor muscles is vital for conducting appropriate pelvic floor exercises. It is possible that activating these muscles in the correct manner might help with the treatment of a variety of pelvic floor issues, as well as sexual health, core stability, and control of the bladder and bowels. In the absence of awareness of these muscles, it is easy to stimulate surrounding muscles such as the glutes, inner thighs, or abdominals, which in turn reduces the effectiveness of exercises that target the pelvic floor.

The Way to Locate the Muscles in Your Pelvic Floor

Identifying your pelvic floor muscles may involve some work, but these simple tactics can help you become more familiar with this vital region of your body.

a. Stopping the Flow of Urine

One of the easiest strategies to identify your pelvic floor muscles is to try to attempt to halt or diminish the flow of pee while using the toilet. If you can successfully halt the stream, you are exercising your pelvic floor muscles. This strategy, however, should only be done for identifying reasons and not as a regular exercise as it could interfere with normal bladder function.

b. Imagine lifting and squeezing.

While sitting comfortably in a chair, maintain your back straight and your feet level with the ground. Close your eyes and image striving to lift a tiny object with the muscles inside your vagina. As you do this, you should feel a gentle squeezing and rising deep inside your pelvis. This exercise helps you to imagine the pelvic floor muscles contracting.

c. Checking for engagement while seated.

Sit on a firm chair or an exercise ball. Keep your legs slightly apart and your feet flat on the floor. Try to lift the area between your pubic bone and tailbone while keeping the rest of your body motionless. You may feel a little stiffness or rising inside your pelvic. This sensation signifies that you're engaging your pelvic floor muscles.

d. Using a Mirror to Provide Visual Feedback

If you feel comfortable doing so, lie down with a hand-held mirror between your legs. When you appropriately tighten your pelvic floor muscles, you may feel a slight lifting or tightness around the vaginal opening. This visual cue may offer quick feedback, which is essential if you are confused whether you are targeting the proper muscles.

e. Using Your Fingers for Self-Examination

Insert a clean, lubricated finger into your vagina and squeeze around it. If you activate the pelvic floor muscles properly, you should notice a mild tightening and lifting sensation. You may try with various positions, such as lying down, sitting, or standing, to see how the experience alters with posture.

f. Applying Biofeedback Devices

Women who fail to detect their pelvic floor muscles on their own may benefit from biofeedback devices. These devices are supposed to monitor muscle activity and offer real-time feedback on whether you're training the proper muscles. Some devices are implanted into the vagina and connect to an app or screen, which leads you through exercises and shows if you've effectively engaged the pelvic floor.

3. Mistakes to Avoid When Identifying Pelvic Floor Muscles

While experimenting with these ways, it's crucial to avoid mistakenly engaging other muscles that can interfere with pelvic floor training:

Avoid Clenching Your Buttocks: Tightening the glutes is a classic blunder that may produce a deceptive appearance of pelvic floor involvement. Concentrate on the internal rising sensation within the pelvis rather than squeezing your buttocks.

Relax Your Inner Thighs: Using the inner thigh muscles could generate erroneous input. Keep your inner thighs relaxed to make sure you're merely working the pelvic floor muscles.

Breathe Naturally: Holding your breath while trying to engage the pelvic floor could place extra strain on the muscles. Practice deep, steady breathing while clenching and releasing your pelvic floor.

4. Practice Makes Perfection.

Learning to identify and isolate the pelvic floor muscles could take some time, especially if they are weak or you've never worked on them before. Spend a few minutes every day utilizing the several tactics outlined above until you feel comfortable identifying and contracting these muscles without engaging other muscle groups.

5. Conducting the 'Lift and Hold' test

Once you're comfortable with your pelvic floor muscles, try the "lift and hold" test to measure your control. To perform this test:

Lie or sit comfortably.

Contract your pelvic floor muscles as if you were trying to lift something inside.

Hold the contraction for 3-5 seconds, breathing slowly.

Gently release the contraction, focussing on the downward and outward movement as you relax.

Try repeating this technique numerous times. If you can contract, hold, and release the pelvic floor muscles without activating other muscles or holding your breath, you've appropriately identified and activated the pelvic floor.

Proper Breathing and Posture

The effectiveness of pelvic floor exercises is directly tied to good breathing and posture. Your breathing and body posture impact how your pelvic floor muscles engage and respond during exercise. Learning appropriate breathing strategies and retaining optimum posture will help you enhance the benefits of pelvic floor exercises, lessen strain, and improve overall pelvic health.

The necessity of good breathing.

Breathing is more than merely an exchange of oxygen; it has a direct influence on the function of the pelvic floor muscles. The diaphragm, the major muscle involved in breathing, communicates with the pelvic floor. When you inhale, your diaphragm moves lower, generating pressure in the abdominal cavity and causing the pelvic floor muscles to stretch. As you exhale, the diaphragm raises, permitting the pelvic floor to lightly compress. When correctly executed, this natural movement enhances the suppleness and strength of the pelvic floor muscles.

How Breath Affects The Pelvic Floor

When you take shallow or rapid breaths with just your chest, the diaphragm and pelvic floor muscles do not work correctly. This may produce needless tension or overactivity in the pelvic floor, especially when paired with poor posture. Deep diaphragmatic breathing (also known as belly breathing) helps the pelvic floor maintain its regular rhythm of contraction and relaxation. Proper breathing habits can promote synchronization of the diaphragm, abdominal muscles, and pelvic floor.

- Help to relax the pelvic floor, alleviating tension and discomfort.
- Increase awareness of pelvic floor muscle movements, resulting in more effective engagement during exercise.
- Reduce intraabdominal pressure, which may lead to pelvic floor dysfunctions like prolapse or incontinence.

Tip: When completing pelvic floor exercises, connect your breathing with muscle contractions. Inhale to prepare and relax the pelvic floor, then exhale while contracting it (similar to a Kegel). This synchronization supports optimal muscle activation while decreasing undesired tension on the pelvic organs.

The Impact of Posture on Pelvic Floor Health.

Posture is another essential aspect in pelvic floor function. The posture of your spine, pelvis, and hips has a direct influence on how your pelvic floor muscles work. Poor posture, such as excessively sagging or arching your lower back, may lessen intra-abdominal pressure and make it harder for the pelvic floor to function effectively.

Optimal posture for pelvic floor workouts.

Achieving good posture distributes pressure equally throughout the body, helping the pelvic floor to adequately support and stabilize the pelvis. Here's how to position oneself for best pelvic floor engagement:

Standing Position: Place your feet hip-width apart, weight evenly distributed between both feet. Maintain a tiny bend in your knees and avoid closing them. Your pelvis should be neutral, not tilted forward (creating an excessive arch in the lower back) or backward (resulting in a tucked tailbone). Softly contract your abdominal muscles to stabilize your spine, then place your head over your shoulders, ears in line with your shoulders.

Seated Position: When sitting, find a firm chair that supports your hips. Place your feet firmly on the floor and sit with your back straight, shoulders relaxed, and ears aligned with your shoulders. Make sure your pelvis is neutral, and your sit bones (the bones at the bottom of your pelvis) are equally planted on the chair. Avoid sagging or bending your lower back, which may strain the pelvic floor.

Lying Down put: When lying down, particularly for pelvic floor exercises, bend your knees and put your feet flat on the floor, hip width apart. Maintain a neutral posture with a slight natural curve in your lower back. Relax your shoulders while maintaining your neck long and aligned with your spine. This position lowers tension on the pelvic floor and assists in the isolation of muscles during exercise.

4. Combined Breathing and Posture

By combining diaphragmatic breathing and appropriate posture, you may create an ideal environment for your pelvic floor to perform effectively. Here's how to bring them together:

Seated Exercise: Sit in a chair with a neutral pelvis and feet flat on the floor. Put your hands on your abdomen. Inhale deeply, expanding your abdomen and allowing your pelvic floor muscles lengthen. Exhale softly, engaging your pelvic floor muscles by gently drawing them upward while preserving your upright posture. Repeat numerous times to relate your breathing to pelvic floor movement.

Standing Exercise: Place your feet hip-width apart, spine neutral. Inhale to relax and expand your pelvic floor muscles. Exhale slowly, lifting and engaging the pelvic floor to keep your spine and pelvis in alignment. To achieve optimum muscle activation, repeat this during routine activities such as walking or bending.

5. Practice Makes Perfection.

Proper breathing and posture require constant practice. As you establish this foundation, it will become easy to incorporate into your normal life and training program. This combination not only increases pelvic floor health, but it also improves overall body mechanics, core stability, and physical well-being.

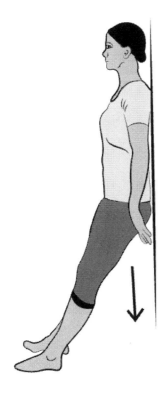
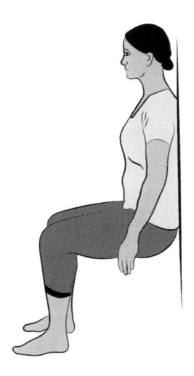

CHAPTER THREE

Basic Pelvic Floor Exercises

Basic Kegel Exercises

Why It Works

Kegel exercises focus to strengthen the muscles of the pelvic floor, which supports the pelvic organs, helps manage the bladder, and improves sexual health.

Goal

To contract and relax the pelvic floor muscles, building strength and endurance for better pelvic support.

How to Do It

1. Sit or lie down in a comfortable position.
2. Take a deep breath, release it, and tense your pelvic floor muscles slightly as if you're halting the flow of urine.
3. Hold the contraction for 3-5 seconds, then slowly release and relax for another 5 seconds.
4. Repeat 10-15 times, gradually increasing the duration of the hold as you build strength.

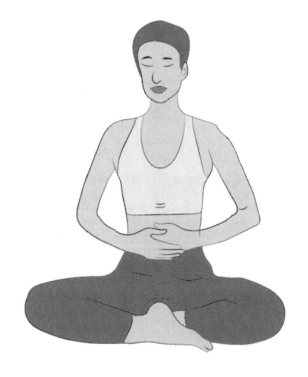

Modification

If holding the contraction for 5 seconds is difficult, start with shorter holds (2-3 seconds) and gradually increase as your muscles strengthen.

Knee to Chest Stretch

Why It Works

This stretch helps relieve tension in the lower back and hips, promoting relaxation of the pelvic floor muscles.

Goal

To gently stretch the lower back, hips, and pelvic region, improving flexibility and reducing muscle tension.

How to Do It

1. Get into a lying down position with your knees bent and your feet planted firmly on the ground.
2. Draw both knee towards your chest, holding them with both hands.
3. Inhale deeply, and as you exhale, gently pull the knees closer to your chest while keeping your lower back pressed into the floor.
4. The stretch should be held for fifteen to thirty seconds as you take deep breaths.
5. Release gradually.
6. Repeat 3-5 times.

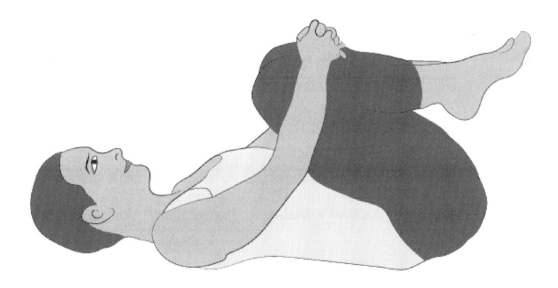

Modification

If pulling the knees close is uncomfortable, use a yoga strap or towel around your thigh to assist in the stretch without straining or consider pulling them one after the oter.

Bridge Pose

Why It Works

Bridge Pose strengthens the glutes, lower back, and pelvic floor muscles, promoting better core stability, posture, and circulation in the pelvic area.

Goal

To engage and strengthen the pelvic floor and glute muscles, supporting proper pelvic alignment and core stability.

How to Do It

1. Lie on your back with knees bent, feet hip-width apart, and arms by your sides.
2. Inhale deeply. As you let your breath out, gently lift the muscles that are located in the pelvic floor.
3. Press your heels into the floor and lift your hips, forming a straight line from knees to shoulders.
4. Hold for 3-5 breaths, maintaining pelvic floor engagement.
5. Slowly lower your hips back down.
6. Repeat 8-10 times.

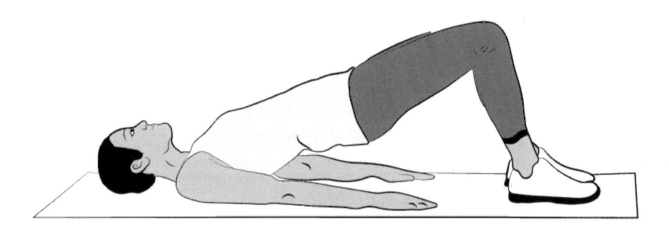

Modification

If lifting your hips fully is difficult, place a pillow or yoga block under your lower back for support.

Pelvic Tilts

Why It Works

Pelvic tilts help strengthen the lower back and core while promoting flexibility and gentle engagement of the pelvic floor muscles.

Goal

To gently activate the pelvic floor muscles, improve pelvic alignment, and enhance lower back flexibility.

How to Do It

1. You should be lying on your back with your knees bent, your feet planted firmly on the ground, and your arms at your sides.
2. Inhale, allowing your belly to rise. As you exhale, flatten your lower back against the floor by tilting your pelvis upward.
3. After holding the tilt for two to three seconds, return to the beginning position and relax.
4. Repeat 10-15 times.

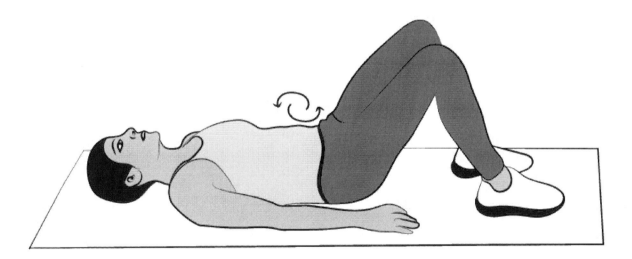

Modification

If lying on your back is uncomfortable, try doing this exercise while seated on a firm chair.

Seated Kegels

Why It Works

Seated Kegels provide an easy way to practice pelvic floor strengthening in a comfortable position, aiding in improved muscle control and endurance.

Goal

To contract and relax the pelvic floor muscles while seated, building strength and muscle awareness.

How to Do It

Position yourself in a comfortable chair with your feet planted firmly on the ground and your back straight.

Inhale deeply. As you exhale, slowly tighten your pelvic floor muscles, as if you are stopping the flow of urine.

Hold the contraction for 3–5 seconds before releasing and relaxing for 5 seconds.

Repeat 10-15 times.

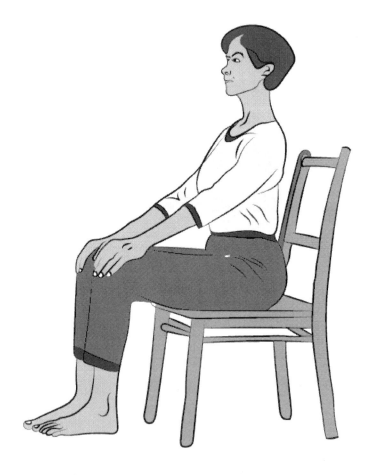

Modification

If holding the contraction is challenging, start with shorter holds (2-3 seconds) and gradually increase as your strength improves.

Standing Kegels

Why It Works

Standing Kegels strengthen the pelvic floor muscles in an upright position, mimicking everyday movements and improving bladder control and core stability.

Goal

To contract and relax the pelvic floor muscles while standing, enhancing muscle strength and endurance.

How to Do It

1. Stand with your feet hip-width apart, knees slightly bent, and hands resting on your hips.
2. Inhale deeply. As you exhale, gently contract your pelvic floor muscles, as if stopping the flow of urine.
3. Hold the contraction for 3–5 seconds before releasing and relaxing for 5 seconds.
4. Repeat 10-15 times.

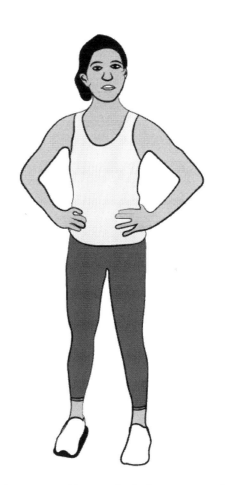

Modification

If you have trouble maintaining balance, rest your hands on a wall or a chair for support. You can also place a pillow in between your leg to increase the contraction.

Supine Hip Rolls

Why It Works

Supine hip rolls help mobilize the lower back and pelvis, gently engaging and relaxing the pelvic floor muscles to improve flexibility and coordination.

Goal

To gently stimulate and rest the pelvic floor and lower back muscles, promoting pelvic balance and movement.

How to Do It

1. You should be lying on your back with your knees bent, your feet planted firmly on the ground, and your arms at your sides.
2. Inhale, allowing your belly to rise. As you exhale, slightly tilt your hips upward, lowering your lower back against the floor.
3. Slowly roll your hips from side to side, keeping your feet and shoulders grounded.
4. Repeat this rolling motion 10-15 times, focusing on the gentle movement of your pelvis.

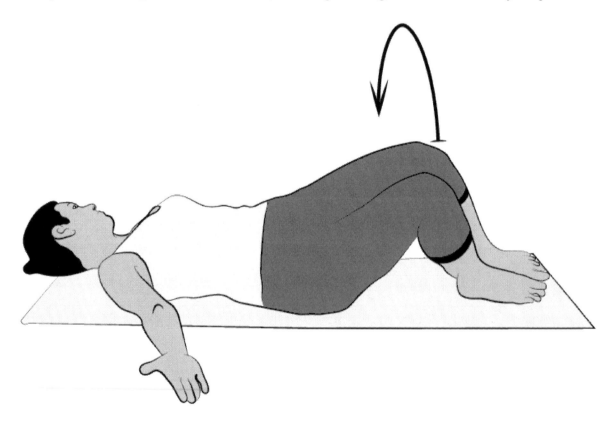

Modification

If the rolling motion feels too intense, reduce the range of motion to small, gentle tilts.

Diaphragmatic Breathing

Why It Works

Diaphragmatic breathing helps relax the pelvic floor, reducing tension and promoting better coordination between the diaphragm and pelvic floor muscles.

Goal

To practice deep breathing that encourages pelvic floor relaxation and enhances core stability.

How to Do It

Place your hands on your abdomen as you comfortably sit or lie down.

Inhale deeply through your nose, allowing your belly to rise and your pelvic floor to relax naturally.

Exhale slowly through your mouth, feeling the pelvic floor gently contract and lift.

Repeat for five to ten breaths, paying attention to your abdomen's rise and fall.

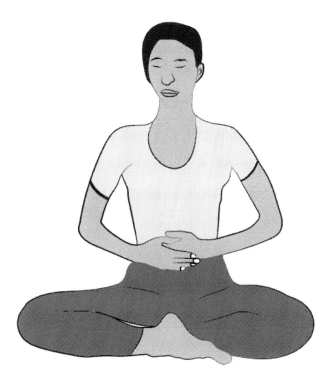

Modification

If lying flat is uncomfortable, try this exercise in a seated or reclined position with your back supported.

Deep Squats

Why It Works

To improve pelvic alignment and strength, deep squats work the glutes, core muscles, and pelvic floor.

Goal

To strengthen the pelvic floor and lower body muscles while improving hip flexibility.

How to Do It

1. With your toes pointed slightly outward, place your feet shoulder-width apart.
2. Inhale deeply, engaging your core and pelvic floor muscles.
3. Exhale as you lower your hips down into a deep squat, keeping your back straight and chest lifted.
4. After three to five seconds of holding the pose, push through your heels to stand again.
5. Repeat 8-10 times.

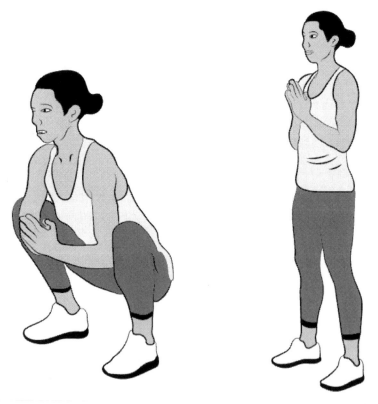

Modification

If full squats are difficult, place a chair behind you and squat down to sit lightly on it before standing back up.

Wall Sits with Pelvic Engagement

Why It Works

Wall sits target the pelvic floor, glutes, and thighs, promoting endurance and stability in the pelvic region.

Goal

To strengthen the pelvic floor and lower body muscles while maintaining proper alignment.

How to Do It

1. Stand with your back against a wall, feet shoulder-width apart, and slide down into a seated position with knees at a 90-degree angle.
2. Inhale, then exhale and gently engage your pelvic floor muscles as if lifting them inward and upward.
3. Hold this position and pelvic engagement for 5-10 seconds, breathing steadily.
4. Slowly slide back up the wall to the starting position.
5. Repeat 8-10 times.

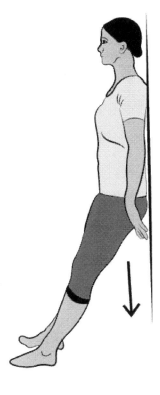 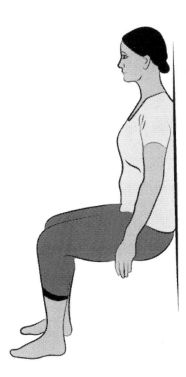

Modification

If holding a full wall sit is too challenging, slide only partway down the wall, reducing the depth of the squat.

CHAPTER FOUR

Intermediate Exercises for Building Pelvic Strength

Chair Pose (Utkatasana)

Why It Works

Chair Pose engages the pelvic floor, thighs, and core muscles, building strength and stability in the lower body while promoting pelvic alignment.

Goal

To strengthen the pelvic floor, thighs, and core while improving balance and posture.

How to Do It

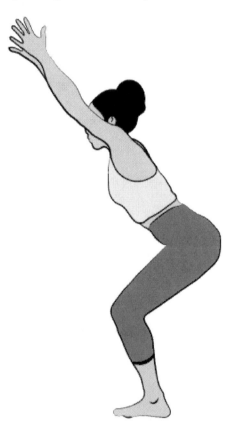

1. Stand with feet hip-width apart, Place your arms at your sides.
2. Inhale, raising your arms overhead.
3. Exhale and bend your knees, dropping your hips as if sitting back into a chair.
4. Engage your pelvic floor muscles as you hold the pose for 5-10 seconds, keeping your knees aligned with your toes.
5. As you stand back up, take a breath.
6. Repeat 8-10 times.

Modification

If balance is challenging, hold onto a chair or wall for support.

Warrior II Pose

Why It Works

Warrior II opens the hips and strengthens the pelvic floor, legs, and core, improving overall stability and muscle control.

Goal

To engage the pelvic floor while strengthening the legs, hips, and core.

How to Do It

1. Stand with feet wide apart, turning your right foot out 90 degrees and left foot slightly inward.
2. Inhale as you lift your arms to shoulder height, keeping them parallel to the floor.
3. Breathe out as you bend your right knee so that it is positioned over your right ankle, while keeping your hips facing outward.
4. Engage your pelvic floor muscles and hold the pose for 5-10 seconds.
5. Inhale as you straighten your right leg, then switch sides.
6. Repeat 5-8 times on each side.

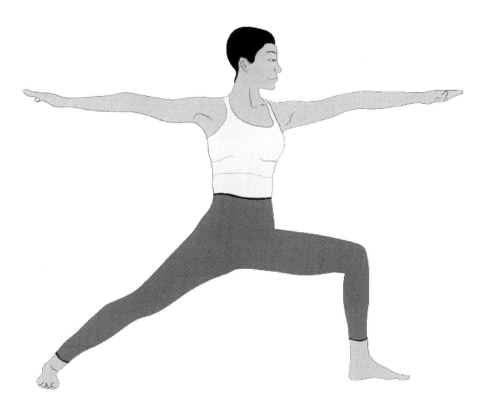

Modification

If maintaining balance is difficult, shorten your stance or rest your back against a wall.

Single-Leg Deadlifts

Why It Works

Single-leg deadlifts activate the pelvic floor, hamstrings, and glutes, improving balance, coordination, and lower body strength.

Goal

To strengthen the pelvic floor, glutes, and hamstrings while enhancing balance.

How to Do It

1. Stand with feet hip-width apart, Place your arms at your sides.
2. Transfer your body's weight to your right leg while maintaining a slight bend in the knee.
3. Inhale as you hinge forward from your hips, lifting your left leg straight back while keeping your back flat.
4. Engage your pelvic floor and core muscles as you lower your torso parallel to the floor.
5. As you come back to the initial position, breathe out and lower your left leg.
6. Repeat 8-10 times on each leg.

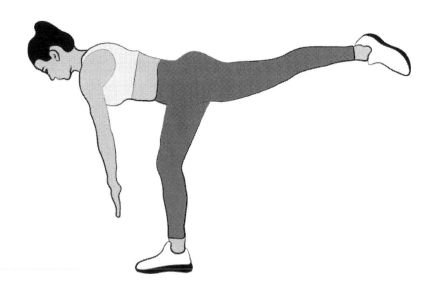

Modification

If balance is a challenge, hold onto a chair or wall for support.

Glute Bridge with Resistance Band

Why It Works

Adding a resistance band to the glute bridge increases the engagement of the pelvic floor, glutes, and hips, building strength and enhancing muscle endurance.

Goal

To strengthen the pelvic floor, glutes, and hip muscles while improving pelvic stability.

How to Do It

1. Place a resistance band just above your knees and lie on your back with your knees bent, feet flat on the floor hip-width apart.
2. As you breathe in, push your knees against the resistance band while breathing out, activating your pelvic floor muscles.
3. Raise your hips up toward the ceiling, creating a straight line from your shoulders to your knees.
4. Hold for 3-5 seconds, then lower your hips back to the floor.
5. Repeat 10-12 times.

RESISTANCE BAND

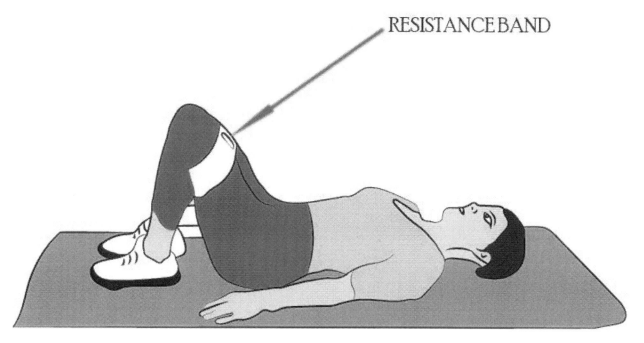

Modification

If the resistance band is too challenging, perform the bridge without the band until you build strength.

Standing Pelvic Circles

Why It Works

Standing pelvic circles improve pelvic floor flexibility, strengthen the core, and enhance coordination, promoting better control and mobility in the pelvic region.

Goal

To activate and relax the pelvic floor and core muscles, enhancing pelvic stability and flexibility.

How to Do It

1. Stand and make sure your feet are positioned shoulder-width apart and place your hands on your hips.

2. Inhale, gently engaging your core and pelvic floor.

3. Circle your hips in a slow motion to the right, and then to the left, creating big, smooth circles.

4. Complete 10 circles in one direction, then switch to the other direction.

Modification

If standing is uncomfortable, perform smaller pelvic circles while seated on a stability ball.

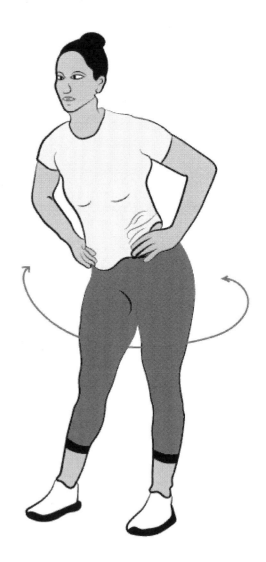

Side-Lying Clamshells

Why It Works

Clamshells target the glutes, hips, and pelvic floor, improving muscle strength and coordination in the lower body.

Goal

To strengthen the glutes, hips, and pelvic floor muscles while enhancing pelvic stability.

How to Do It

1. Lie on your side with knees bent at a 90-degree angle and your legs stacked.
2. Inhale, engaging your pelvic floor and core. As you exhale, lift your top knee toward the ceiling, keeping your feet together.
3. Hold your knee up for 2-3 seconds, then gradually bring it back down.
4. Repeat 10-12 times on each side.

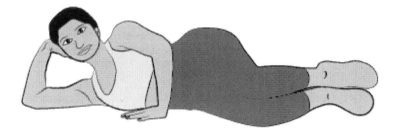

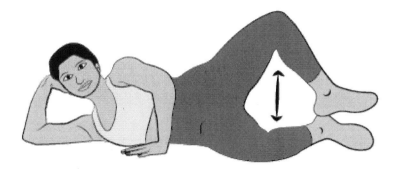

Modification

If possible, perform the clamshells with resistance band to gain more strength.

Wide-Legged Forward Fold

Why It Works

This particular stretch is beneficial for easing tension in the pelvic floor and hamstrings, which encourages flexibility and relaxation in the pelvic area.

Goal

To lengthen and relax the pelvic floor muscles while stretching the inner thighs and hamstrings.

How to Do It

1. Stand with your feet wider than shoulder-width apart, toes pointing slightly forward.
2. Inhale deeply, lengthening your spine.
3. Exhale and slowly hinge at your hips, folding forward and reaching your hands toward the floor.
4. Place your hands on the ground or on a yoga block for support. Hold onto the position for 15-30 seconds while taking deep breaths.
5. Slowly return to a standing position by engaging your core and pelvic floor as you rise.

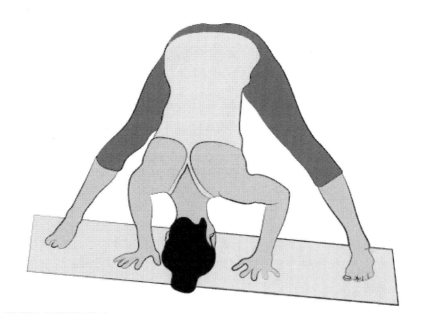

Modification

When you experience tightness in the hamstrings or lower back, consider bending your knees slightly for added comfort.

Lateral Lunges

Why They Work

Lateral lunges work the pelvic floor, glutes, and inner thighs, strengthening and stabilizing the lower body.

Goal

Strengthen the pelvic floor, glutes, and thighs while increasing hip mobility and balance.

How To Do It

1. Place your hands on your hips or put them in a prayer position and stand with your feet hip-width apart.
2. Inhale and take a big stride to the right, bending your right knee but maintaining your left leg straight.
3. Exhale and push through your right heel to return to the starting posture.
4. Throughout the activity, keep your pelvic floor muscles engaged.
5. Repeat eight to ten times on each side.

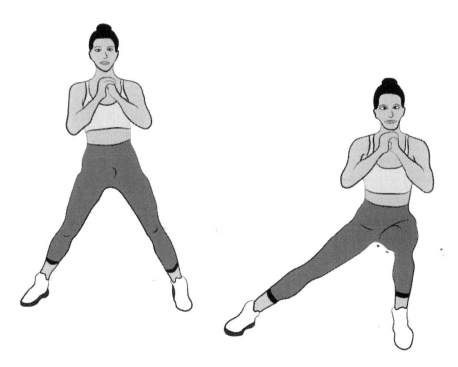

Modification

If balance is difficult, grip onto a chair or a wall for support while doing the lunge.

Reverse Lunges

Why It Works

Reverse lunges work the glutes, hamstrings, and pelvic floor, increasing lower-body strength and stability while improving balance.

Goal

To strengthen the pelvic floor, glutes, and thighs while improving balance and control.

A

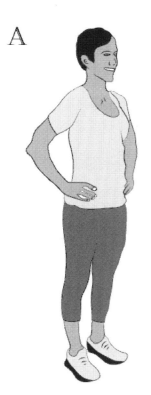

How To Do It

1. Stand hip-width apart, hands on hips.
2. Inhale, then step your right foot back into a lunge, bending both knees to form a 90-degree angle.
3. As you sink into the lunge, softly contract your pelvic floor muscles.
4. Exhale and push your front heel back to the beginning position.
5. Repeat 8 to 10 times on each leg.

B

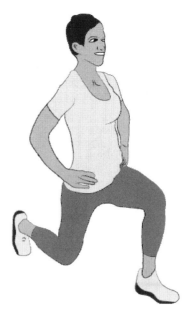

Modification

If keeping balance is difficult, grip onto a chair or a wall for support while doing the lunges.

Frog Pumps

Why They Work

Frog pumps strengthen the glutes and activate the pelvic floor, so stabilizing the pelvis and increasing muscular endurance.

Goal

To stimulate and develop the pelvic floor and gluteus muscles while improving pelvic stability.

How To Do It

1. Lie on your back, knees bent and feet together, and let your knees fall outward into a **"frog"** stance.
2. Inhale, then exhale while pressing your feet together and lifting your hips to the sky.
3. Squeeze your glutes and engage your pelvic floor at the apex of the exercise.
4. Lower your hips back to the ground and repeat.
5. Perform 12 to 15 repetitions.

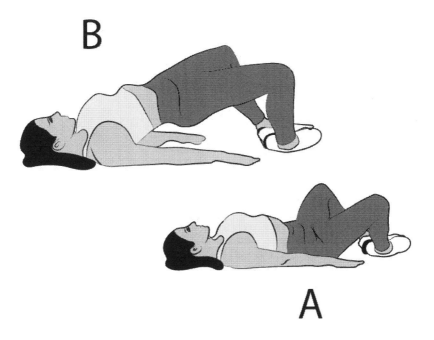

Modification

If raising your hips is difficult, lay a cushion or yoga block behind your lower back for more support.

CHAPTER FIVE

Advanced Pelvic Strength Exercises

Standing Hip Abduction with Resistance Bands

Why it works

This exercise improves the pelvic floor, glutes, and outer thighs, resulting in increased hip stability and lower body strength.

Goal

To strengthen the pelvic floor and gluteus muscles while improving hip stability.

How To Do It

1. Place a resistance band around your ankles and stand hip-width apart.

2. Engage the core and pelvic floor muscles.

3. Slowly raise your right leg out to the side while keeping it straight and resisting the band.

4. Before going back to the starting position, hold for two to three seconds.

5. Repeat ten to twelve times on each leg.

Modification

If keeping balance is difficult, hang onto a chair or a wall for support while doing the exercise.

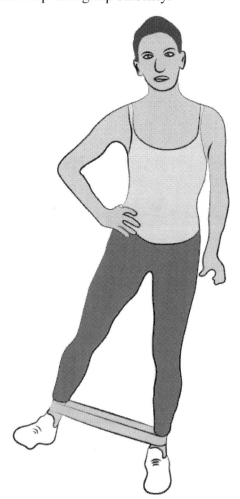

Squat Pulses with Small Exercise Ball

Why it works

Squat pulses with a tiny exercise ball improve lower-body strength, endurance, and muscular control.

Goal

To strengthen the pelvic floor, glutes, and thighs while increasing lower-body endurance.

How To Do It

1. Position a small exercise ball between your thighs and stand with your feet hip-width apart.
2. Inhale, then drop into a squat posture, gently gripping the ball between your thighs to stimulate the pelvic floor.
3. Pulse up and down in tiny motions while holding the ball between your legs.
4. Perform 15-20 pulses while maintaining pelvic floor engagement.

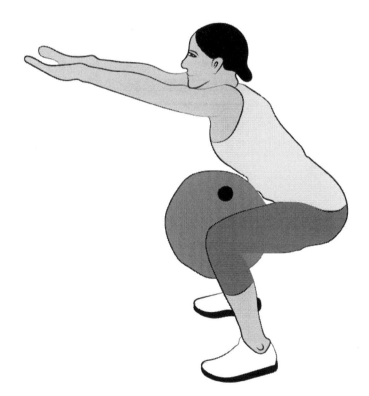

Modification

If squatting low is problematic, use shallow pulses to decrease knee strain and gradually increase strength.

Modified Side Plank with Hip Drop

Why it works

This exercise works the pelvic floor, obliques, and glutes, increasing core stability and pelvic strength.

Goal

Strengthen the pelvic floor, core, and hip muscles while increasing endurance and stability.

How To Do It

1. Lie on your side, forearms supporting your upper body, knees bent.
2. Engage your core and pelvic floor, then raise your hips off the ground into a side plank.
3. Slowly drop your hip towards the floor without touching it, then raise it back to its original position.
4. Repeat eight to ten times on each side.

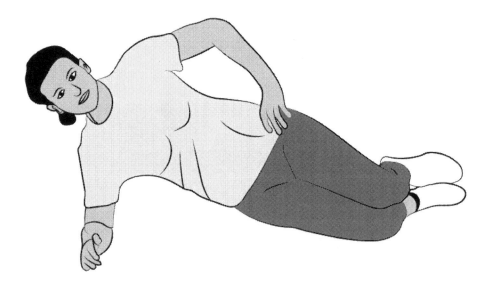

Modification

If this is too difficult, maintain the side plank posture without hip dips and concentrate on pelvic floor engagement.

Tabletop Leg Extensions

Why They Work

Tabletop leg extensions help to strengthen the pelvic floor, core, and glutes, which improves stability and coordination.

Goal

Engage the pelvic floor and core muscles while improving balance and control.

How To Do It

1. Begin on all fours in a tabletop posture, with your hands under your shoulders and knees under your hips.
2. Inhale, then activate your core and pelvic floor.
3. Keep your right leg straight back and your hips level.
4. Before going back to the starting position, hold for two to three seconds.
5. Alternate legs, doing 10-12 extensions on each side.

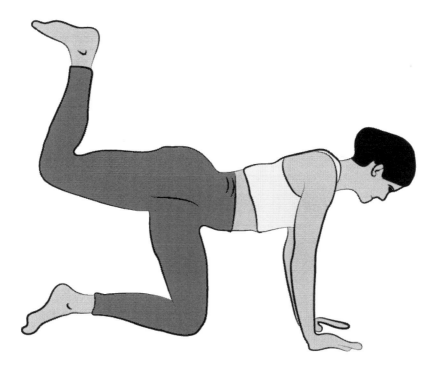

Modification

If balance is difficult, keep the toes of the extended leg barely contacting the floor for extra support.

Bridge Pose with Single-Leg Lift

Why it works

This advanced version of the bridge position works the pelvic floor, glutes, and hamstrings, improving pelvic stability and lower-body strength.

Goal

Strengthen the pelvic floor and glute muscles while increasing single-leg balance and control.

How To Do It

1. Lie on your back, knees bent, feet hip-width apart.
2. Inhale. As you exhale, squeeze through your heels and raise your hips into the bridge pose.
3. Engage your pelvic floor and core, then raise your right leg off the floor and stretch it straight out.
4. Hold for 3-5 seconds, then return your leg and hips to their starting position.
5. Repeat 8 to 10 times on each leg.

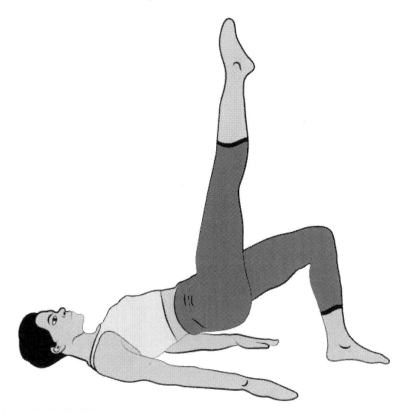

Modification

If raising a leg proves too difficult, maintain both feet on the ground and execute a basic bridge stance until you have adequate strength.

Fire Hydrant Exercise

Why it Works

The fire hydrant exercise works the glutes, hips, and pelvic floor, which improves hip mobility, strength, and pelvic stability.

Goal

Strengthen the pelvic floor, glutes, and hips while increasing hip stability and coordination.

How To Do It

1. Begin on all fours in a tabletop posture, with your hands under your shoulders and knees under your hips.
2. Engage your core and pelvic floor.
3. Lift your right leg out to the side until it is hip height while keeping your knee bent.
4. Hold for 2-3 seconds, then gently drop your leg back to its original position.
5. Repeat ten to twelve times on each side.

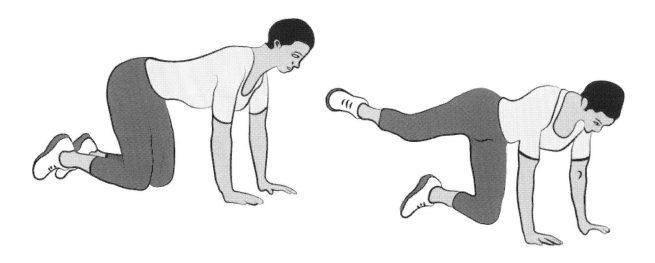

Modification

If this is too difficult, do smaller leg lifts to decrease hip strain until you gain strength.

Frog Jumps

Why It Works

Frog jumps are a high-intensity workout that works the pelvic floor, glutes, and thighs, building strength, endurance, and explosive power.

Goal

Strengthen the pelvic floor, glutes, and legs while increasing power and cardiovascular endurance.

How To Do It

1. Stand with your feet wider than shoulder width apart and toes pointed outward.
2. Lower yourself into a deep squat, with your hands on the floor between your feet.
3. Explosively leap forward, landing lightly in a squat stance.
4. Jump forward again, keeping the pelvic floor and core engaged.
5. Perform 8-10 leaps per set.

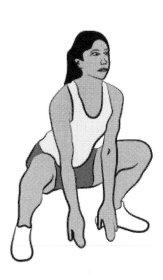
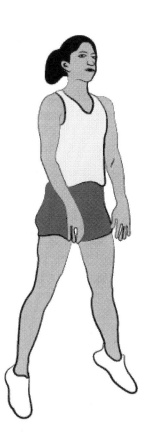

Modification

If leaping is too strenuous, try deep squats in position, concentrating on pelvic floor engagement.

Warrior III Pose

Why It Works.

Warrior III improves the pelvic floor, glutes, legs, and core while also improving balance and stability.

Goal

Engage the pelvic floor and core muscles while increasing lower body strength and balance.

How To Do It

1. Stand with your feet hip-width apart, then move your weight to your right leg.
2. Inhale while engaging your core and pelvic floor. As you exhale, lean forward at the hips and raise your left leg straight back.
3. Extend your arms forward while maintaining a straight line from your fingers to your elevated heel.
4. Hold for 5-10 seconds with your hips level and pelvic floor engaged.
5. Slowly return to your starting posture and swap legs.
6. Repeat 5–8 times on each leg.

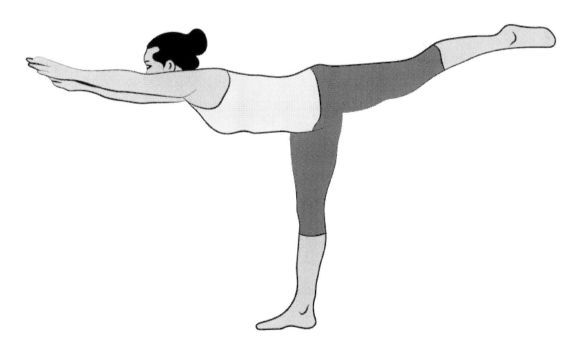

Modification

If balance is difficult, put your hands on a wall or a chair for support while lifting your leg.

Boat Pose (Navasana)

Why it works

Boat Pose with Leg Extensions works the pelvic floor, core, and hip flexors, improving core strength and pelvic stability.

Goal

To improve the pelvic floor, core, and hip muscles while increasing muscular endurance.

How To Do It

1. Sit on the floor, knees bent, feet flat. Put your hands behind your thighs for support.
2. Inhale while engaging your core and pelvic floor. As you exhale, raise your feet off the floor and balance on your sit bones.
3. Extend your legs straight out, maintaining your back straight and your chest up.
4. Hold for 5-10 seconds, then return your knees to their initial position.
5. Repeat 8 to 10 times.

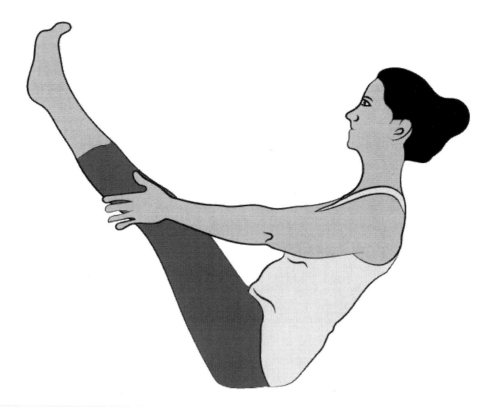

Modification

If extending both legs is difficult, keep your knees bent and alternate between extending one leg at a time for extra assistance.

CHAPTER SIX

Exercises for Postpartum Recovery

Reclined Deep Belly Breathing

Why it works

Deep belly breathing helps the pelvic floor and core muscles reconnect after birth, increasing calm and muscular control.

Goal

To relax the pelvic floor, enhance breath control, and gradually activate the core muscles.

How To Do It

1. Lie on your back, bend your legs and place your feet flat on the ground.
2. Put a hand on your chest or beside you and another on your stomach.
3. Take a deep breath in through your nostrils while stretching your abdominal muscles and keeping your chest in a stable position.
4. The exhalation should be done slowly through the lips, with the intention of softly stimulating your pelvic floor and bringing your belly button closer to your spine.
5. Repeat for 5 to 10 breaths, concentrating on relaxation and mild engagement.

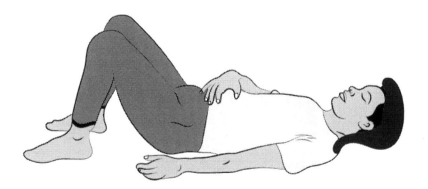

Modification

If lying flat is unpleasant, use cushions to support your back and neck.

Supine heel slides

Why They Work.

Heel slides strengthen the lower abdominal muscles and pelvic floor, which improves core strength and pelvic stability.

Goal

Gently activate the pelvic floor and lower abdominal muscles while improving pelvic control.

How To Do It

1. Lie on your back, bend your legs and place your feet flat on the ground.

2. Inhale deeply. As you exhale, contract your pelvic floor and gradually pull one heel away from your body until your leg is straight.

3. Inhale as you move your heel back to its starting position.

4. Alternate legs, doing 8-10 slides on each side.

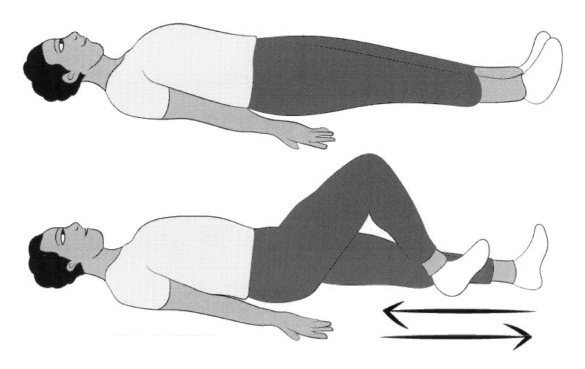

Modification

If this proves too difficult, slip the heel halfway before returning to the starting position.

Seated Marching

Why it Works

Seated marching softly works the pelvic floor, hip flexors, and core muscles, resulting in better muscular control and stability.

Goal

Strengthen the pelvic floor and core while increasing coordination and balance.

How To Do It

1. Sit erect in a chair, feet flat on the floor, hands resting on your thighs.
2. Inhale while activating your pelvic floor and core muscles.
3. Exhale as you pull your left knee to your chest while maintaining your back straight.
4. Return your left foot to the floor and repeat with the right leg.
5. Alternate legs, doing 10-12 marches on each side.

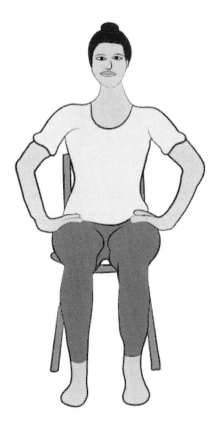 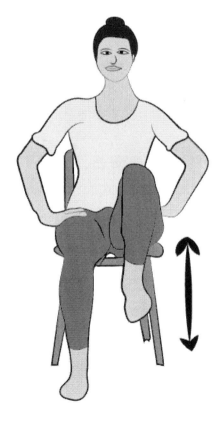

Modification

If elevating the knee high proves difficult, begin with tiny, moderate lifts until you gain strength.

Side-Lying Leg Lifts

Why They Work

Side-lying leg raises work the glutes, hips, and pelvic floor, which helps to develop pelvic strength and stability.

Goal

Strengthen the pelvic floor, glutes, and hips while increasing hip stability and control.

How To Do It

1. Lie on your side, legs stacked, knees straight.
2. Support your head with your lower arm and place your upper hand on the floor in front of you to keep your equilibrium.
3. Inhale while activating your pelvic floor and core muscles.
4. Exhale as you elevate your upper leg to hip height while maintaining it straight.
5. Hold for 1-2 seconds before gently lowering your leg back down.
6. Do 8-10 repetitions on each side.

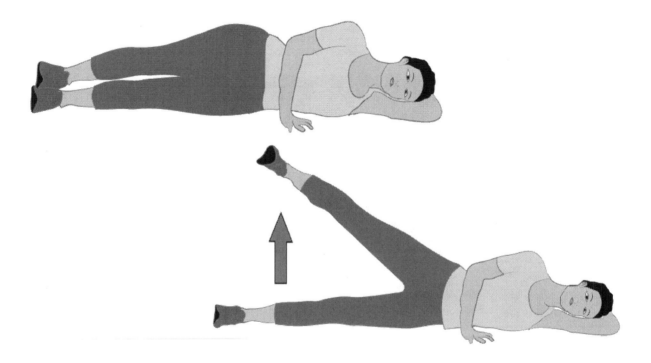

Modification

If elevating your leg completely is difficult, bend your knees slightly to limit your range of motion.

Modified Bird Dog

Why it works

The modified bird-dog exercise works the pelvic floor, core, and glutes, enhancing stability and balance while reducing lower-back pain.

Goal

To strengthen the pelvic floor, core, and glutes while improving coordination and stability.

How To Do It

1. Start in a tabletop position on all fours, placing your knees behind your hips and your wrists beneath your shoulders.
2. Inhale while activating your pelvic floor and core.
3. Exhale gently, extending your right arm forward and your left leg straight back while maintaining your hips level.
4. Before going back to the starting position, hold for two to three seconds.
5. Alternate sides, repeating 8-10 times on each side.

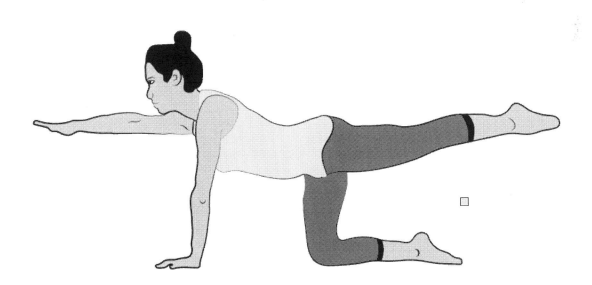

Modification

If extending both the arm and the leg is too difficult, begin by extending either the arm or the leg until you gain strength and balance.

Butterfly Stretch

Why It Works

The butterfly stretch opens the hips and gently stretches the pelvic floor, encouraging relaxation and suppleness in the pelvis.

Goal

To relieve stress in the pelvic floor and inner thighs, which improves flexibility and blood flow.

How To Do It

1. With your feet together, legs bowed, and back straight, take a seat on the floor.
2. Hold your feet with both hands, allowing your knees to fall outward.
3. Inhale deeply, then exhale as you gently push your knees to the floor, experiencing a stretch in your inner thighs.
4. For 15 to 30 seconds, hold the stretch while inhaling deeply.

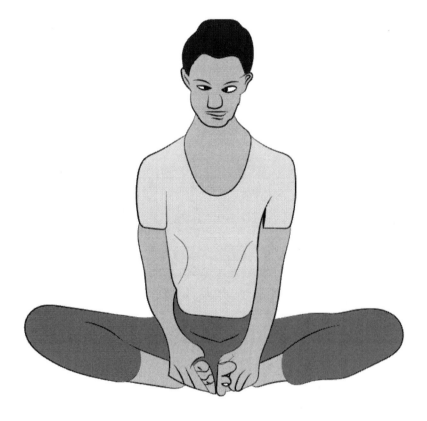

Modification

If this stretch is too difficult, lay cushions beneath your knees to provide additional support and comfort.

Supine Core Activation with Small Ball or Pillow

Why It Works.

This workout employs a tiny ball or pillow to engage the core and pelvic floor muscles, hence enhancing muscular awareness and control.

Goal

Engaging the pelvic floor and deep core muscles improves pelvic stability and muscular strength.

How To Do It

1. Lie on your back with your knees bent and your feet level on the floor. Place a small ball or pillow between your knees.
2. Inhale deeply. As you exhale, gently grasp the ball or pillow with your knees to activate your inner thighs and pelvic floor muscles.
3. Bring your belly button towards your spine at the same time to activate your core.
4. After three to five seconds of holding the contraction, release it.
5. Repeat 10 to 12 times.

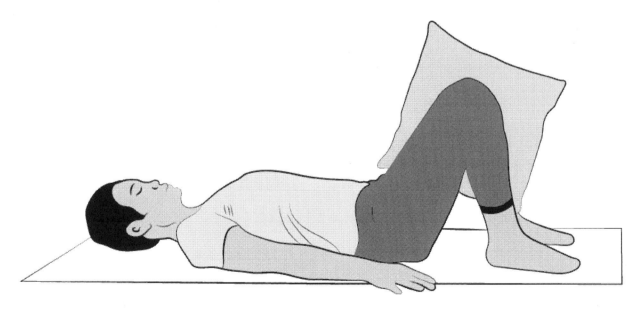

Modification

If squeezing the ball proves difficult, try a soft cushion or folded cloth for a gentler activation.

Gentle squats (without weights)

Why it works

Gentle squats help to strengthen the pelvic floor, glutes, and thighs while also improving lower-body balance and flexibility.

Goal

To strengthen the pelvic floor and leg muscles while maintaining pelvic alignment.

How To Do It

1. Place your feet shoulder width apart, toes pointing slightly outward.
2. Inhale, then gently bend your knees, lowering your hips into a squat posture with your back straight.
3. Exhale and push through your heels to return to a standing posture, activating your pelvic floor as you rise.
4. Repeat 8-10 times with a calm, controlled motion.

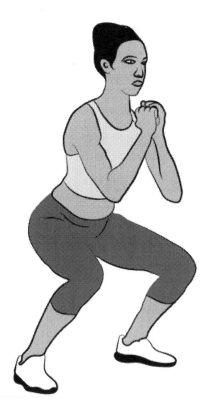

Modification

If squatting deeply is difficult, set a chair behind you and crouch down to gently touch it before rising up.

CHAPTER SEVEN

Exercises to Manage Incontinence

Quick Flick Kegels

Why It Works

Quick Flick Kegel exercises use fast contractions to target the pelvic floor muscles, enhancing muscular reactivity and control for managing abrupt impulses.

Goal

To swiftly activate and strengthen the pelvic floor muscles, hence preventing leaks produced by unexpected pressure, such as sneezing or coughing.

How To Do It

1. Sit or lay in a comfortable posture.
2. Inhale deeply. As you exhale, swiftly clench your pelvic floor muscles to halt the flow of pee.
3. Immediately release and relax.
4. Perform fast contractions, aiming for ten quick flicks in succession.
5. Rest for a few seconds, then repeat the set 2-3 times.

Modification

If quick contractions are problematic, begin with slower flicks and then increase the pace as your pelvic floor muscles strengthen.

Seated Kegels with a Small Ball Squeeze

Why They Work

Combining Kegels with a tiny ball squeeze increases resistance, allowing the pelvic floor muscles to be strengthened more efficiently for incontinence management.

Goal

To increase pelvic floor strength, use both the pelvic and inner thigh muscles simultaneously.

How To Do It

1. Sit in a chair, feet flat on the floor, and put a tiny ball between your knees.
2. Inhale, then exhale and gently grasp the ball with your knees, squeezing your pelvic floor muscles.
3. Hold the pressure for 3–5 seconds before relaxing.
4. Repeat 10 to 12 times.

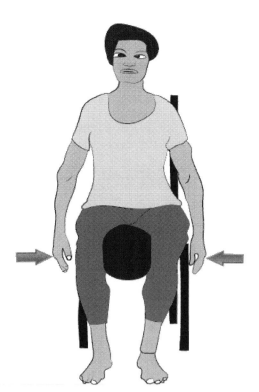

Modification:

If holding the squeeze is difficult, add a soft pillow or cushion for milder resistance.

Hip Bridges with Inner Thigh Squeeze

Why it Works

This exercise strengthens the pelvic floor, glutes, and inner thighs, resulting in improved bladder control and pelvic organ support.

Goal

To activate the pelvic floor and inner thighs while strengthening the glutes and increasing pelvic stability.

How To Do It

1. Lie on your back with your knees bent and your feet level on the floor. Put a little ball between your knees.
2. Inhale deeply. As you exhale, grasp the ball with your knees to activate your inner thighs and pelvic floor muscles.
3. Make a straight line from your shoulders to your knees and push through your heels to lift your hips off the ground if possible.
4. After three to five seconds of holding the position, drop your hips once again.
5. Repeat 10 to 12 times.

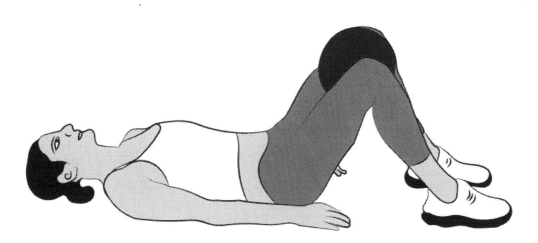

Modification

If raising your hips completely is difficult, do the bridge without the ball and concentrate on a mild pelvic lift.

Supine Marching

Why It Works

This exercise gently activates the pelvic floor and core, helping improve muscle control and pelvic stability.

Goal

To strengthen the pelvic floor and core muscles while enhancing coordination and stability.

How to Do It

1. Get into a lying down position with your knees bent and your feet planted firmly on the ground.
2. Inhale, engaging your pelvic floor and core muscles.
3. Exhale as you slowly lift your right foot off the floor, bringing your knee toward your chest.
4. Lower your foot back to the starting position and repeat with the left leg.
5. Alternate legs, performing 8-10 marches on each side.

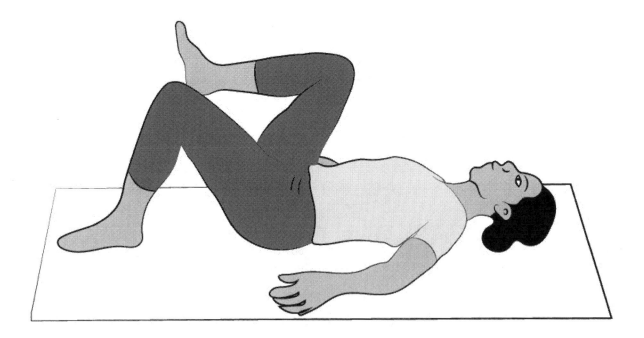

Modification

If lifting the leg high is challenging, start with smaller movements, only raising the foot a few inches off the ground.

CHAPTER EIGHT

Exercises To manage pelvic pain

Child's Pose (Balasana)

Why it works

Child's Pose softly stretches the lower back, hips, and pelvic floor, which promotes relaxation and relieves pelvic tension.

Goal

To relieve stress in the pelvic floor and lower back, hence improving relaxation and flexibility.

How To Do It

1. Begin on your hands and knees, big toes together and knees apart.
2. Sit back on your heels and stretch your arms forward, bringing your forehead to the floor.
3. Inhale deeply, feeling your belly rise and your pelvic floor relax.
4. Hold this posture for 30 seconds to 1 minute, breathing deeply and concentrating on relaxation.

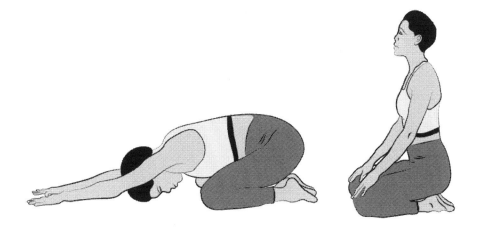

Modification

If you are experiencing difficulty, place a cushion or blanket behind your knees or between your hips and heels for extra support.

Happy baby pose (Ananda Balasana)

Why it works

Happy Baby Pose softly stretches the inner thighs, hips, and pelvic floor, which helps to relieve stress and promote pelvic flexibility.

Goal

Stretching and releasing tension from the pelvic floor and hip muscles promotes relaxation.

How To Do It

1. Bring your knees up to your chest while lying on your back.
2. Hold the outside borders of your feet with your hands and allow your knees to bend and open toward your armpits.
3. Inhale deeply, releasing your pelvic floor and letting your hips expand.
4. Hold for 30 seconds to 1 minute, swaying side to side as desired.

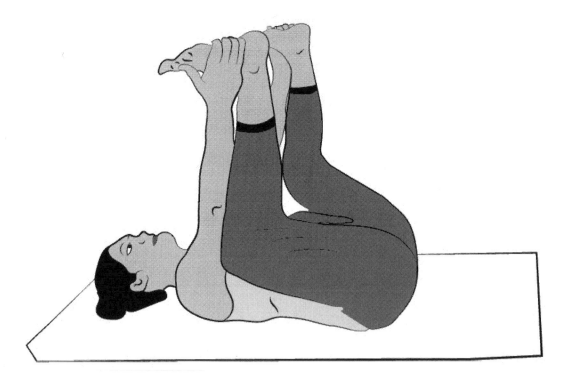

Modification

If it is difficult to reach your feet, grab your shins or wrap a yoga strap over each foot for support.

Seated Forward Fold

Why it works

Seated Forward Fold stretches the hamstrings and lower back, helping to relax the pelvic floor and relieve pelvic tension.

Goal

Stretching the lower back, hamstrings, and pelvic floor muscles increases flexibility and reduces stress.

How To Do It

1. You should be seated on the floor with your legs in front of you in a straight line.
2. Inhale while sitting tall and stretching your spine.
3. Exhale and gently bend at the hips, bringing your hands to your feet while maintaining your back straight.
4. Continue to hold the stretch for twenty to thirty seconds while taking deep breaths and allowing your pelvic floor to relax.

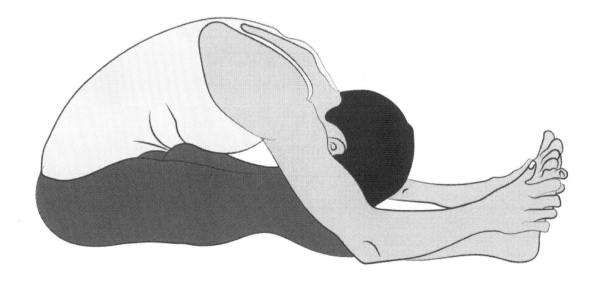

Modification:

Place a yoga strap over your feet or bend your knees slightly to alleviate tension on the hamstrings and lower back.

Reclined Bound Angle Pose

Why It Works

This posture opens the hips and extends the inner thighs, which helps to reduce tension and promote relaxation in the pelvic floor.

Goal

Stretching the inner thighs and pelvic floor promotes relaxation and suppleness in the pelvis.

How To Do It

1. Lie on your back, knees bent.
2. The soles of your feet should be brought together, and you should allow your knees to fall to the sides.
3. Put your hands by your sides or on your stomach. Inhale deeply and concentrate on relaxing your pelvic floor.
4. Hold the posture for one to two minutes, inhaling slowly and deeply.

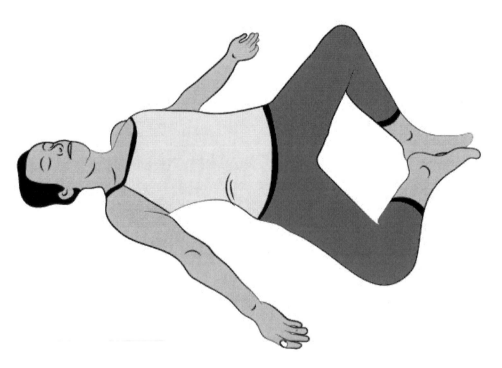

Modification

If your hips are tense, use cushions or folded blankets beneath your knees for support.

Cat-Cow Stretch

Why it works

The Cat-Cow Stretch softly mobilizes the spine and pelvis, which helps to release tension in the pelvic floor and lower back.

Goal

Enhance pelvic and spinal mobility by relaxing and releasing tension in the pelvic floor.

How To Do It

1. Begin on all fours, placing your wrists beneath your shoulders and your knees under your hips.
2. Inhale as you arch your back (Cow Pose), raising your tailbone and head while lowering your tummy.
3. Exhale and curve your spine (Cat Pose), tucking your tailbone and moving your belly button closer to your spine.
4. Continue to move between these two postures for 8-10 calm breaths.

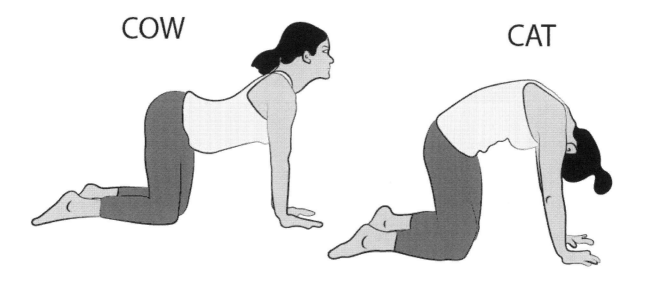

Modification

If kneeling is difficult, tuck a folded blanket between your knees to provide more padding.

Hip Flexor Stretch

Why It Works

The hip flexor stretch relaxes the hips and pelvis, which helps to reduce pelvic floor stiffness and increase flexibility.

Goal

To stretch the hip flexors and gradually relieve tension in the pelvic floor, hence improving pelvic mobility.

How To Do It

1. Begin in a kneeling lunge stance, right foot forward and left knee on the floor.
2. Place your hands on your right knee for support, then slowly press your hips forward while maintaining your upper body erect.
3. Inhale deeply and feel a stretch at the front of your left hip.
4. Hold for 20-30 seconds, then go to the opposite side.

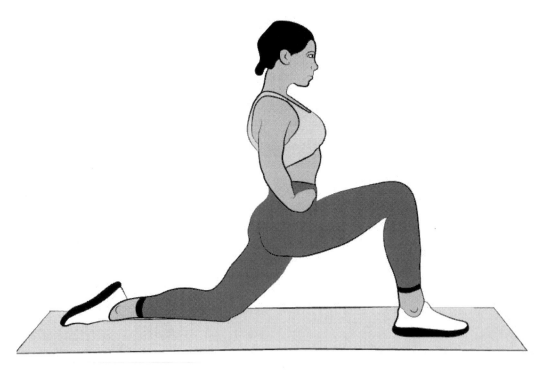

Modification

If kneeling is unpleasant, lay a folded blanket beneath your knee to provide more support.

Supine Twist (supta matsyendrasana)

Why it works

This twist softly stretches the lower back and hips, relaxing the pelvic floor and increasing spinal flexibility.

Goal

Stretching the lower back and hips aids in alleviating pelvic tension and encourages relaxation.

How To Do It

1. Get into a lying down posture, knees bent and feet firmly planted on the ground.

2. Extend your arms to the sides in a "T" posture.

3. Inhale, then exhale, gently lowering your knees to the right while maintaining your shoulders planted.

4. Hold for 20-30 seconds while inhaling deeply.

5. Inhale as you return your knees to center, then repeat on the left side.

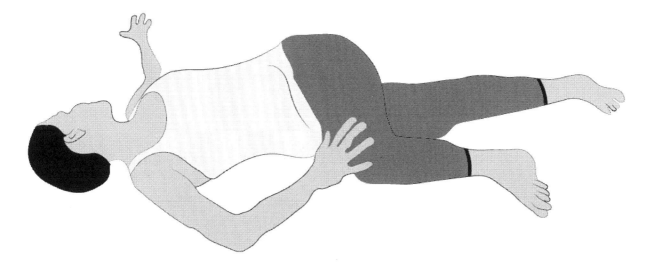

Modification

Place a cushion or blanket under your knees for support if the twist is too strong.

Reclined Pigeon Pose

Why It Works

Reclined Pigeon Pose stretches the hips, glutes, and lower back, which helps to relieve pelvic floor tension and promote relaxation.

Goal

Stretching the hip muscles and glutes reduces pelvic stress and increases flexibility.

How To Do It

1. Get into a laying down posture, knees bent and feet firmly planted on the ground.
2. Make a "4" form by crossing your right ankle over your left knee.
3. Gently raise your left foot off the ground and grasp the back of your left leg with both hands.
4. Inhale deeply, then exhale as you bring your left leg toward your chest, feeling the stretch in your right hip.
5. Hold for 20-30 seconds and then swap sides.

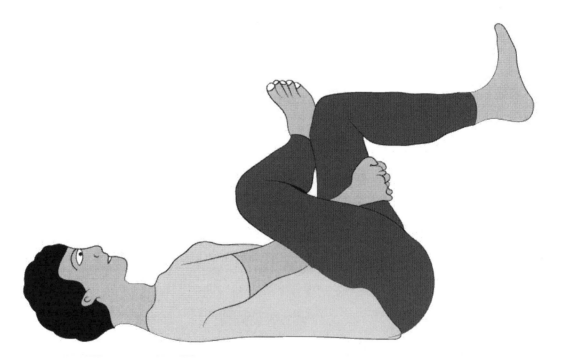

Modification

Keep your left foot planted on the floor and gently push your right knee away from your body if lifting the leg toward your chest is too difficult.

Seated Spinal Twist

Why It Works.

The sitting spinal twist stretches the spine, hips, and pelvis, producing relaxation and increased pelvic mobility.

Goal

To improve pelvic mobility and flexibility while reducing hip and lower back tension.

How To Do It

1. Sit on the floor, legs outstretched.
2. Place your right foot on the outside of your left leg and bend your right knee.
3. For support, place your right hand on the ground behind you.
4. Inhale and stretch your spine. Place your left elbow on the outside of your right knee and exhale as you turn your body to the right.
5. Before swapping sides, hold the twist for 20 to 30 seconds.

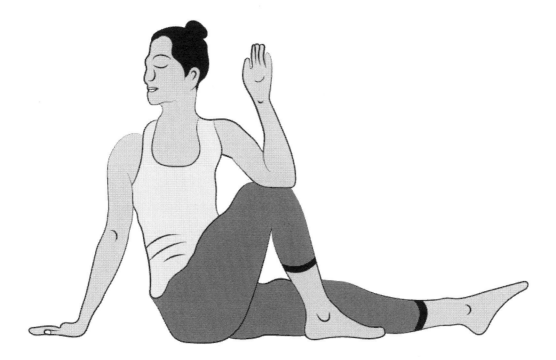

Modification

If sitting with both legs extended causes discomfort, keep your left leg bent and your foot on the floor for further support.

Legs Up the Wall Pose

Why it works

Legs-Up-the-Wall Pose promotes relaxation and increases circulation in the pelvic region, which helps to relieve pelvic floor stress and pain.

Goal

To relax the pelvic floor, increase blood flow, and relieve stress in the lower body.

How To Do It

1. One side of your body should be seated against a wall.
2. With your hips close to the wall, drop your head and back to the floor and swing your legs gently up the wall.
3. With your palms facing up, place your arms at your sides.
4. Take a deep breath and relax your pelvic floor.
5. Hold this stance for three to five minutes, inhaling gently and deeply.

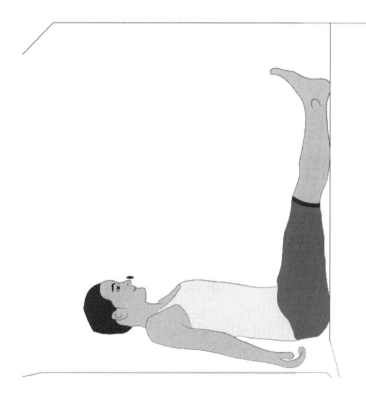

Modification

If sleeping flat makes you uncomfortable, place a folded blanket or pillow beneath your hips for added support.

CHAPTER NINE

Pelvic Floor Release and Strengthening Exercises.

Garland pose (Malasana)

Why it works

Garland Pose is a deep squat that opens the hips and extends the pelvic floor, which helps to relieve stress and strengthens the pelvic area.

Goal

Stretching the hips, lower back, and pelvic floor improves flexibility and relieves stress in the pelvis.

How To Do It

1. Stand with your feet slightly wider than hip-width apart and toes pointed outward.
2. Inhale deeply, then exhale while bending your knees and lowering your hips into a deep squat.
3. Bring your hands together at your chest, then squeeze your elbows into your inner knees to increase the stretch.
4. Hold for 20–30 seconds, taking a deep breath and focusing on pelvic floor relaxation.

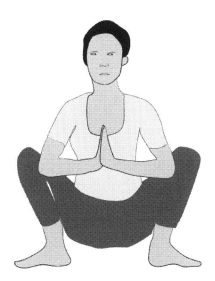

Modification

If squatting deeply is difficult, lay a wrapped blanket or yoga block under your heels for support.

Hand-to-Big-Toe Pose

Why Does It Work?

This position stretches the hamstrings, hips, and pelvic floor, which promotes pelvic tension relief and flexibility.

Goal

Stretch the hamstrings and hips while releasing tension in the pelvic floor.

How To Do It

1. Lie on your back, legs outstretched.
2. After taking a breath, bend your right knee and bring it close to your chest.
3. Place a yoga strap or a rolled towel over the arch of your right foot and gently straighten your leg, stretching it toward the sky.
4. Hold for 20-30 seconds while inhaling deeply. Switch sides.

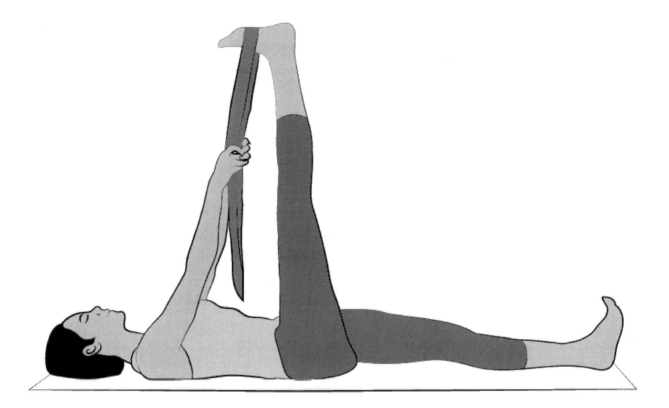

Modification

If you can't reach your foot, bend your knee slightly and use a towel instead of a yoga strap.

Pigeon pose

Why it works

Pigeon Pose stretches the hips, glutes, and lower back, which helps to relieve deep tension in the pelvic floor and surrounding muscles.

Goal

Stretching the hips and glutes will help to relieve pelvic stiffness and strain.

How To Do It

1. Begin on all fours. Bring your right knee forward and position it behind your right wrist, then stretch your right ankle toward your left wrist.
2. Slide your left leg back, straightening the knees and lowering your hips to the floor.
3. Inhale deeply to stretch your spine. Exhale, then gradually drop your body over your right leg, resting on your forearms or forehead.
4. Hold for 20-30 seconds and then swap sides.

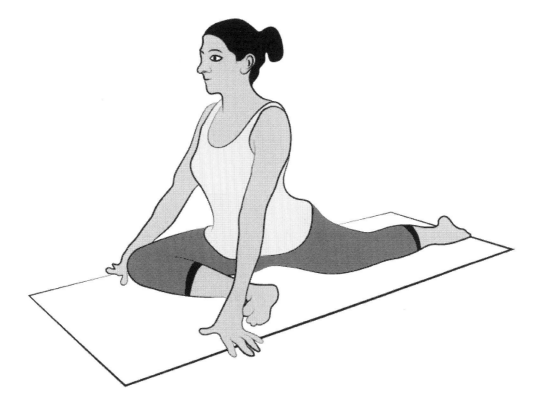

Modification

If this posture is too challenging, tuck a folded blanket or pillow under your right hip for support.

Goddess Pose (Utkata Konasana)

Why It Works

Goddess Pose improves the pelvic floor, inner thighs, glutes, and core, hence improving pelvic stability and muscular endurance.

Goal

To work the pelvic floor, thighs, and glutes while developing balance and lower body strength.

How To Do It

1. Stand with your feet wide apart and toes pointed slightly outward.
2. Inhale deeply. As you exhale, bend your knees and drop into a squat while maintaining your back straight.
3. Bring your arms to a "goalpost" position (elbows bent at 90 degrees) and squat for 20-30 seconds while breathing deeply.
4. To return to standing, engage your pelvic floor and inner thigh muscles by pressing through your feet.

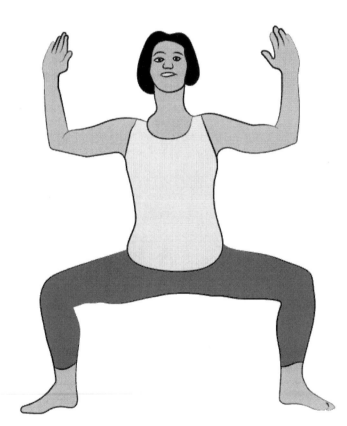

Modification

If balance is difficult, execute the squat with your back against a wall for more support.

Camel pose (Ustrasana)

Why it works

Camel Pose stretches the front body, particularly the hips, pelvic floor, and abdomen, which promotes pelvic release and increases flexibility.

Goal

Stretching the hip flexors, abdomen, and pelvic floor muscles helps to improve release and posture.

How To Do It

1. Kneel on the floor, hip-width apart, and place your hands on your lower back for support.
2. Inhale deeply to elevate your chest and stretch your spine.
3. Exhale as you softly lean back, putting your hands to your heels or resting them on your back for support.
4. Hold for 15-30 seconds, inhaling deeply and letting your pelvis and chest expand.

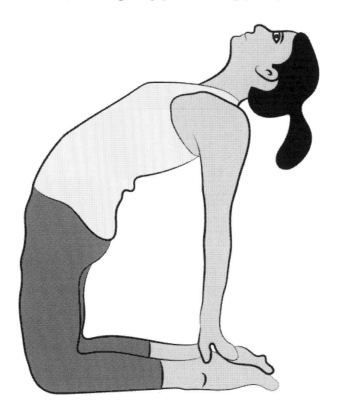

Modification

If reaching your heels is tough, tuck your toes under to elevate them or rest your hands on your lower back for support.

Tree Pose (Vrksasana) with Pelvic Floor Awareness

Why It Works

Tree Pose enhances balance and stability by activating the pelvic floor and core, fostering awareness and gradual strengthening of the pelvic region.

Goal

To strengthen the pelvic floor and core muscles while increasing balance and coordination.

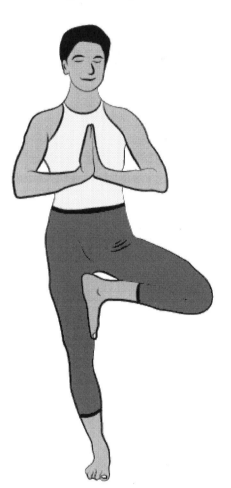

How To Do It

1. Stand upright, positioning your feet at hip-width and letting your arms rest comfortably at your sides.
2. Shift your weight to your right leg and place the sole of your left foot on your inner right thigh or calf.
3. Place your hands at your heart or reach them up high to help find your balance.
4. Inhale deeply, then exhale while engaging your pelvic floor and holding your balance for 20-30 seconds.
5. Switch sides.

Modification

If balance is difficult, lean your back against a wall or keep your toes on the ground for more support.

CHAPTER TEN

28-DAY WORKOUT PLAN

Here's an organized 4-week, 28-day workout schedule that builds from basic to intermediate workouts, using exercises from each chapter of this book. This program includes strength training, pelvic floor release, and targeted recovery and incontinence exercises. Every day begins with a warm-up, followed by main exercises and a cool-down.

Week 1: Foundational Strength and Awareness

Day 1

Warm-up: Diaphragmatic Breathing (3 mins)

Main Exercises:

- Basic Kegel Exercises (3 sets of 10 reps)
- Knee to Chest Stretch (2 sets of 20 seconds per side)
- Bridge Pose (3 sets of 10 reps)

Cool-down: Supine Hip Rolls (2 sets of 10 reps)

Day 2

Warm-up: Deep Squats (2 sets of 10 reps)

Main Exercises:

- Pelvic Tilts (3 sets of 10 reps)
- Seated Kegels (3 sets of 10 reps)
- Wall Sits with Pelvic Engagement (3 sets of 20 seconds)

Cool-down: Knee to Chest Stretch (1 set of 30 seconds per side)

Day 3

Rest Day: Focus on deep breathing

Day 4

Warm-up: Deep Squats (2 sets of 10 reps)

Main Exercises:

- Standing Kegels (3 sets of 10 reps)
- Seated Kegels with a Small Ball Squeeze (3 sets of 10 reps)
- Supine Marching (2 sets of 10 reps)

Cool-down: Child's Pose (1 set of 30 seconds)

Day 5

Warm-up: Diaphragmatic Breathing (3 mins)

Main Exercises:

- Bridge Pose (3 sets of 10 reps)
- Knee to Chest Stretch (2 sets of 20 seconds per side)
- Butterfly Stretch (1 set of 30 seconds)

Cool-down: Seated Forward Fold (1 set of 30 seconds)

Day 6

Warm-up: Diaphragmatic Breathing (3 mins)

Main Exercises:

- Quick Flick Kegels (3 sets of 10 reps)
- Supine Heel Slides (3 sets of 10 reps)

- Seated Marching (2 sets of 10 reps)

Cool-down: Cat-Cow Stretch (1 min)

Day 7

Rest Day: Gentle walk and breathing exercises

Week 2: Introducing Intermediate Strength Building

Day 8

Warm-up: Supine Core Activation with Small Ball (2 sets of 10 reps)

Main Exercises:

- Chair Pose (Utkatasana) (3 sets of 10 seconds)
- Glute Bridge with Resistance Band (3 sets of 10 reps)
- Side-Lying Clamshells (3 sets of 10 reps per side)

Cool-down: Child's Pose (1 min)

Day 9

Warm-up: Supine Marching (2 sets of 10 reps)

Main Exercises:

- Wide-Legged Forward Fold (2 sets of 15 seconds)
- Standing Pelvic Circles (2 sets of 15 seconds per side)
- Lateral Lunges (3 sets of 8 reps per side)

Cool-down: Happy Baby Pose (1 min)

Day 10

Rest Day: Deep breathing exercises and gentle stretches

Day 11

Warm-up: Supine Core Activation with Small Ball (2 sets of 10 reps)

Main Exercises:

- Single-Leg Deadlifts (3 sets of 8 reps per side)
- Reverse Lunges (3 sets of 8 reps per side)
- Frog Pumps (3 sets of 10 reps)

Cool-down: Cat-Cow Stretch (1 min)

Day 12

Warm-up: Diaphragmatic Breathing (3 mins)

Main Exercises:

- Wall Sits with Pelvic Engagement (3 sets of 20 seconds)
- Butterfly Stretch (2 sets of 30 seconds)

- Seated Forward Fold (1 set of 30 seconds)

Cool-down: Supine Twist (1 min)

Day 13

Warm-up: Seated Spinal Twist (1 min per side)

Main Exercises:

- Warrior II Pose (3 sets of 10 seconds per side)
- Side-Lying Leg Lifts (3 sets of 10 reps per side)
- Frog Pumps (3 sets of 10 reps)

Cool-down: Happy Baby Pose (1 min)

Day 14

Rest Day: Walk and focus on deep breathing

Week 3: Progressing to Advanced Movements

Day 15

Warm-up: Supine Pelvic Clock Exercise (1 min)

Main Exercises:

- Standing Hip Abduction with Resistance Band (3 sets of 10 reps per side)
- Squat Pulses with Small Exercise Ball (3 sets of 10 reps)
- Modified Side Plank with Hip Drop (3 sets of 8 reps per side)

Cool-down: Child's Pose (1 min)

Day 16

Warm-up: Cat-Cow Stretch (1 min)

Main Exercises:

- Chair Pose (Utkatasana) (3 sets of 10 seconds)
- Wide-Legged Forward Fold (2 sets of 15 seconds)
- Side-Lying Clamshells (3 sets of 10 reps per side)

Cool-down: Supine Twist (1 min)

Day 17

Rest Day: Gentle stretches

Day 18

Warm-up: Supine Core Activation (1 min)

Main Exercises:

- Tabletop Leg Extensions (3 sets of 10 reps per side)
- Fire Hydrant Exercise (3 sets of 10 reps per side)
- Reverse Lunges with Pelvic Engagement (3 sets of 8 reps per side)

Cool-down: Reclined Bound Angle Pose (1 min)

Day 19

Warm-up: Diaphragmatic Breathing (3 mins)

Main Exercises:

- Glute Bridges with Resistance Band (3 sets of 10 reps)

- Modified Side Plank with Kegel Hold (3 sets of 10 seconds per side)
- Squats with Pelvic Floor Engagement (3 sets of 10 reps)

Cool-down: Legs-Up-the-Wall Pose (1 min)

Day 20

Warm-up: Deep breathing

Main Exercises:

- Warrior III Pose (3 sets of 10 seconds per side)
- Frog Jumps (3 sets of 8 reps)
- Seated Marching (2 sets of 10 reps)

Cool-down: Happy Baby Pose (1 min)

Day 21

Rest Day: Focus on relaxation exercises

Week 4: Strength and Release Focus

Day 22

Warm-up: Supine Pelvic Clock Exercise (1 min)

Main Exercises:

- Garland Pose (3 sets of 10 seconds)
- Warrior II Pose with Pelvic Engagement (3 sets of 10 seconds per side)
- Glute Bridge with Resistance Band (3 sets of 10 reps)

Cool-down: Child's Pose (1 min)

Day 23

Warm-up: Butterfly Stretch (1 min)

Main Exercises:

- Bridge Pose with Single-Leg Lift (3 sets of 10 reps per side)
- Seated Forward Bend (1 min hold)
- Fire Hydrant Exercise (3 sets of 10 reps per side)

Cool-down: Reclined Bound Angle Pose (1 min)

Day 24

Rest Day: Light stretching

Day 25

Warm-up: Diaphragmatic Breathing (3 mins)

Main Exercises:

- Boat Pose (Navasana) with Leg Extensions (3 sets of 10 seconds)
- Frog Jumps (3 sets of 8 reps)
- Standing Kegels (3 sets of 10 reps)

Cool-down: Reclined Pigeon Pose (1 min)

Day 26

Warm-up: Cat-Cow Stretch (1 min)

Main Exercises:

- Goddess Pose (3 sets of 10 seconds)
- Tree Pose with Pelvic Floor Awareness (3 sets of 10 seconds per side)
- Squat Pulses with Small Exercise Ball (3 sets of 10 reps)

Cool-down: Legs-Up-the-Wall Pose (1 min)

Day 27

Warm-up: Supine Core Activation (1 min)

Main Exercises:

- Camel Pose (3 sets of 10 seconds)
- Glute Bridge with Resistance Band (3 sets of 10 reps)
- Modified Bird Dog (3 sets of 10 reps per side)

Cool-down: Supine Twist (1 min)

Day 28

Rest Day: Relaxation and reflection

Each week builds on the previous, encouraging gradual progress from basic awareness to more advanced strengthening, balancing, and relaxation techniques.

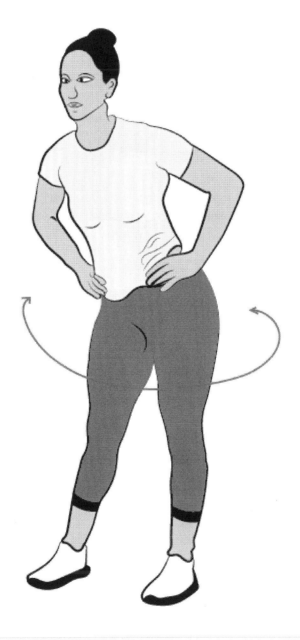

CHAPTER ELEVEN

Frequently Asked Questions (FAQs)

1. How can I tell if my pelvic floor muscles are weak?

Identifying weak pelvic floor muscles may be difficult since symptoms vary greatly. Urinary leaks (particularly when sneezing, coughing, or exercising), bowel control difficulties, a feeling of heaviness or pressure in the pelvic area, and decreased sexual pleasure or sensitivity are also common symptoms. Some women report lower back discomfort or struggle to hold in gas. It is important to highlight that pelvic floor weakness is not limited to elderly women; many young women and new moms have similar symptoms. If you experience these symptoms, it might be an indication that your pelvic floor muscles need to be strengthened, and simple pelvic exercises are an excellent place to start. However, if symptoms continue or worsen, visit a pelvic health expert for an examination.

2. How long will it be before I see results?

The time it takes to notice improvements from pelvic floor exercises varies depending on the person and muscle strength level at the start. Most individuals report significant gains after 4-6 weeks of continuous practice. Subtle effects, such as improved bladder control or less back pain, may be seen within the first few weeks, but complete results might take up to three months. Consistency is essential here; everyday practice, even in short sessions, reinforces these improvements. As you continue to develop your pelvic muscles, you may notice that your posture, core stability, and overall body awareness improve.

3. Can I overdo pelvic floor exercises?

The pelvic floor, like any other muscular area, may be overused. Excessive exercise or poor technique may result in a hypertonic (overly tight) pelvic floor, causing pain, discomfort, and even urine retention. Muscle pain, weariness in the pelvic region, and tension in surrounding regions such as the lower abdomen and thighs are all signs that you may be performing too many pelvic exercises. Balance is essential; giving muscles time to rest and recuperate allows them to develop stronger without being overworked. Aim to follow the planned plan presented in this book, which progressively develops in intensity, and remember that it is completely OK to take pauses or adjust exercises as necessary.

4. Are Pelvic Floor Exercises Safe during Pregnancy?

In general, pelvic floor exercises are quite advantageous during pregnancy, as they may assist support the expanding uterus, relieve back discomfort, and lower the chance of issues such as prolapse. Strengthening these muscles also prepares the body for labor, as a strong pelvic floor may help during the pushing stage, while flexibility is also important for a smooth delivery. However, since each pregnancy is unique, you should always speak with your obstetrician or midwife before beginning or maintaining any fitness program. They may provide particular advice based on your pregnancy stage and health, ensuring that you remain both safe and active.

5. How Can I Fit Exercise Into a Busy Lifestyle?

One of the benefits of pelvic floor exercises is their versatility—they can be done anywhere and frequently without anybody knowing. Simple exercises, like as seated or standing Kegels, may be performed while sitting at your desk, waiting in line, or driving. If finding a regular time each day is difficult, consider "habit stacking"—placing your pelvic exercises alongside everyday chores such as brushing your teeth, waiting for your morning coffee, or commuting. Set phone reminders to help you remain on track. Remember that consistency, not length, makes the difference. Even brief sessions may be quite helpful when done on a regular basis.

6. What Should I Do If I Feel Pain During Exercise?

Pain during pelvic floor exercises may suggest that your muscles are hyperactive or stiff, or that your form need modification. If you have pain when exercising, stop immediately and check your posture and breathing; often merely altering these components might relieve discomfort. If the discomfort continues, try lowering the intensity of your activity or switching to a milder exercise. Pain may also indicate that you need a more tailored treatment, so contacting a pelvic health professional may be prudent. They may walk you through proper methods and changes to guarantee a safe and productive practice.

7. Will these exercises help my sexual health?

Absolutely. Pelvic floor exercises improve blood flow, flexibility, and muscular control in the pelvis, all of which lead to greater sensitivity, pleasure, and comfort during intimacy. Strengthening these muscles may also help women feel more secure and in control of their bodies, which improves sexual health. Furthermore, a healthy pelvic floor promotes core stability, making movement easier and more pleasant. Whether you're in pain or just want to better your personal life, daily pelvic exercises may result in substantial increases in sensation and enjoyment.

8. How often should I do pelvic floor exercises?

For novices, everyday practice is essential to increase awareness and provide a solid basis. As your muscles are stronger, you may lower the frequency to 3-4 times per week for maintenance. A organized regimen, such as the one described in this book, takes a balanced approach to frequency and intensity. Each person's demands are unique, so if you experience any pain, it's OK to change your regimen or miss a day. Progress is more vital than perfection, and your health will benefit from a consistent, long-term strategy.

9. When Should I See a Health Care Professional?

If you have chronic pain, discomfort, or symptoms that do not improve with regular activity, you should see a healthcare expert. It's also critical to get medical attention if you have diseases such as prolapse, severe incontinence, or other uncommon symptoms that might point to a more serious underlying problem. A pelvic health professional, such as a physiotherapist, may give examinations, personalized instruction, and even physical treatment to help you develop. Remember that it's always best to contact us early to avoid problems from developing and to guarantee that your fitness regimen is both safe and effective.

10. Are Pelvic Floor Exercises Effective for All Ages?

Yes, pelvic floor exercises are useful to women of any age. Younger women often strengthen their pelvic floors to avoid future problems, but older women may concentrate on lowering signs of weakness, such as incontinence or pelvic pain. The workouts in this book are intended to accommodate all fitness levels and may be modified for age or ability. Pelvic floor exercises should be practiced consistently, regardless of age, to increase bladder control, core stability, and overall physical health.

11. Are there any exercises that I should avoid?

Certain exercises might strain the pelvic floor, particularly if you're new to pelvic strengthening or have pre-existing difficulties. High-impact workouts, such as heavy lifting, vigorous sprinting, or high leaping, should be handled with caution since they may put strain on the pelvis. Similarly, any action that causes considerable abdominal strain should be done with caution. Always emphasize workouts that strengthen and stabilize the core and pelvic muscles without producing undue stress.

12. Will I need any equipment to complete this program?

While many pelvic floor exercises just need your body weight, a few programs in this book may include resistance bands, tiny exercise balls, or stability balls to improve engagement and advancement. These tools may provide diversity and challenge as you progress. However, all equipment is optional; you may tailor any workout to your tastes and availability of equipment.

13. How Do Pelvic Floor Exercises Increase Core Strength?

The pelvic floor is an important part of the "core unit," which comprises the deep abdominal muscles, diaphragm, and back muscles. Strengthening the pelvic floor helps to balance the whole region, which improves posture, relieves back discomfort, and makes everyday motions more fluid and controlled. As you develop your pelvic floor, you should experience improved alignment, reduced strain, and a greater sense of body awareness.

14. Do Pelvic Floor Exercises Help with Menopause Symptoms?

Yes, pelvic floor exercises are quite useful in treating some menopausal symptoms, such as urinary incontinence, vaginal dryness, and decreased muscle tone. As estrogen levels drop, pelvic floor strength may gradually reduce, making regular exercise even more important. Pelvic floor exercises serve to offset these effects, providing for increased muscular support and resilience during menopause and beyond.

15. What Is the Best Way to Stay Motivated?

Setting modest, attainable objectives might help maintain motivation over time. Tracking your progress, whether with a diary, a checklist, or a smartphone app, gives visible inspiration as you gain power. Celebrate your progress, no matter how tiny. Consider attending a support group or finding an accountability partner to discuss your experiences. Remember that frequent pelvic floor exercises improve your entire quality of life, and each effort takes you closer to better health and wellbeing.

16. Do Pelvic Floor Exercises Help With Back Pain?

Yes, they often can. A firm pelvic floor supports the lower spine, stabilizing the core and reducing tension on the back muscles. Weak pelvic floor muscles may cause pelvic misalignment or instability, leading to or exacerbating lower back discomfort. As you strengthen the pelvic floor, the muscles that support your spine and posture become more coordinated, putting less pressure on your lower back. Regular pelvic floor exercises, along with core and back exercises, may be extremely effective in relieving or preventing back discomfort.

17. What is the relationship between the pelvic floor and posture?

The pelvic floor helps to maintain healthy posture by supporting the spine with other core muscles. When these muscles are strong and balanced, they serve to stabilise the pelvis, allowing for a neutral spine alignment and adequate weight distribution. Conversely, if the pelvic floor is weak or stiff, it may cause compensatory strain in other regions of the body, including the lower back, hips, and shoulders, resulting in poor posture and pain. Pelvic floor exercises may help improve postural awareness and alignment, making it easier to stand, sit, and move in a balanced and standing up position.

18. Are there exercises for specific pelvic floor issues?

Yes, exercises may be designed to help particular pelvic floor concerns including incontinence, prolapse, or discomfort. For example, quick flick. Kegels may aid with urge incontinence, and simple stretching and relaxation exercises can help with pelvic discomfort caused by muscular stiffness. Those with prolapse may benefit from workouts that strengthen not just the pelvic floor but also the surrounding core muscles, so providing greater support for the pelvic organs. This book is designed to take you through a number of exercises that address various demands, with choices for changing and adapting each activity to meet your own needs.

19. How do I know if I'm doing Kegels correctly?

To conduct Kegels properly, engage and elevate the pelvic floor muscles without squeezing the glutes, thighs, or lower abdomen. To assess your technique, picture halting the flow of pee in the middle (though this should not be done on a frequent basis as it might lead to other problems) or slightly tightening the pelvic muscles as if lifting a tiny item. Instead of a squeeze or clench, you should sense a gentle lift within. If you're uncertain, see a pelvic health professional who can give you feedback and help you establish the proper technique for best outcomes.

20. Can Men Benefit from Pelvic Floor Exercises?

Absolutely. Although this book focuses on women's pelvic health, males may benefit from pelvic floor exercises to improve incontinence, pelvic discomfort, and erectile function. The fundamentals are generally similar, with a focus on strengthening and coordinating the pelvic floor muscles. Pelvic floor exercises may help men maintain prostate health and recuperate from prostate surgery. Anyone interested may modify the exercises in this book to meet their unique requirements or visit resources geared for men's pelvic health.

21. Should I Do Pelvic Floor Exercises If I Am Overweight?

Pelvic floor exercises are useful regardless of weight. In fact, they may be particularly beneficial if you are overweight, since extra weight can put strain on the pelvic floor, perhaps leading to incontinence or prolapse. Strengthening these muscles gives additional support and resilience, allowing you to do everyday tasks more easily. Pelvic floor exercises combined with other types of physical activity, as well as a healthy diet, may improve general health and reduce pressure on the pelvic region.

22. Are There Any Signs That My Pelvic Floor Is Getting Stronger?

Increased bladder control, little or no leakage, and a sense of core stability and support are all signs of progress. Some individuals feel less pelvic or lower back pain and better posture. You may also notice increased body awareness and ease in activating the pelvic floor muscles during exercises. Gradual increases in endurance during exercise, such as being able to hold a Kegel for longer or execute more repetitions, are also indicators of increased pelvic floor strength.

23. What is the purpose of breathing in pelvic floor exercises?

Breathing is essential to pelvic floor exercises. The pelvic floor muscles collaborate closely with the diaphragm, therefore coordinating breath with movement allows the muscles to activate and release effectively. Inhale to enable the diaphragm to descend lower and stretch the pelvic floor, then exhale as you gently raise or activate the pelvic muscles. Proper breathing improves muscular coordination, lowers tension, and increases oxygen flow, so promoting muscle endurance and relaxation. Diaphragmatic breathing, in particular, is an effective approach to improve pelvic floor function and decrease stress.

24. How Do I Prevent Pelvic Floor Dysfunction in the Future?

Consistent pelvic floor exercises, paired with regular physical activity, may help preserve pelvic health throughout life. Additionally, avoiding persistent straining during bowel movements, lifting with right technique, and controlling stress may all help to maintain pelvic floor integrity. Maintaining proper posture and doing core strengthening exercises on a regular basis also help to prevent problems. Maintaining a healthy weight and using good breathing methods might help to relieve unneeded strain on the pelvic floor, minimizing the chance of dysfunction as you age.

25. Can I Do These Exercises After Surgery?

Yes, pelvic floor exercises are often suggested after pelvic-related procedures such as hysterectomy, cesarean birth, or other abdominal surgery. However, you should visit your doctor or a pelvic health therapist for clearance and advice on when to begin. Beginning with easy, low-intensity workouts may help restore muscular strength and flexibility, improving healing while avoiding strain. As your body recovers, you may progressively proceed to more complex workouts to ensure a complete recovery.

26. Are Pelvic Floor Exercises Effective for Constipation Relief?

Yes, pelvic floor exercises, particularly those geared toward relaxation, may help relieve constipation by encouraging more natural bowel movements. Tension in the pelvic floor muscles may interfere with bowel movement, therefore exercises like deep belly breathing, pelvic tilts, and moderate stretches can help release it. Maintaining excellent posture, keeping hydrated, and eating fiber-rich meals may all help with digestive health, in addition to pelvic floor exercises.

27. Is it normal to have soreness after doing pelvic floor exercises?

Mild pain or muscular exhaustion is typical, particularly if you're new to these workouts or increasing the intensity. This is akin to the muscular discomfort you can experience following a new exercise. However, acute pain or lasting discomfort is uncommon and may suggest improper technique or overuse. If discomfort persists, lessen the intensity or frequency of the exercises and visit a pelvic health professional to verify you're doing them safely and successfully.

28 Will Pelvic Floor Exercises Improve My Ability to Exercise and Lift Weights?

Strengthening the pelvic floor helps improve stability and control during physical activity such as lifting, jogging, and other types of exercise. A healthy pelvic floor is part of the core support system, which helps to regulate intra-abdominal pressure and offers a sturdy platform for lifting and movement. As you gain pelvic strength and awareness, you may find it simpler to engage your core and maintain appropriate form, lowering your risk of injury when exercising.

29. Are there any exercises I should avoid if I have a weak pelvic floor?

If you have a weak pelvic floor, you should avoid workouts that exert too much downward pressure on the region, such as heavy lifting, high-impact activities, or severe core exercises (such as crunches or sit-ups), until your pelvic floor strengthens. Exercises that create strain or bulging in the pelvic region should be done with care. Begin with the low-impact, moderate exercises in this book, concentrating on steady development, and work with a healthcare practitioner to adjust high-intensity activities safely.

30. How Can I Include Pelvic Floor Exercises in My Daily Routine?

With a few little tweaks, you may easily include pelvic floor exercises into your everyday regimen. Kegels may be practiced while performing other things like brushing your teeth, commuting, or taking breaks at work. Setting reminders on your phone or integrating workouts into other daily duties may help the pattern become second nature. Consistency is crucial, so scheduling a few minutes of exercise throughout your day may have long-term advantages for your pelvic health.

CONCLUSION

After you've done reading this pelvic floor health guide, take some time to reflect on your experiences. Pelvic floor exercises do more than simply strengthen a set of muscles; they help you restore control, confidence, and resilience in your body. You've made significant steps toward long-term health by learning about the anatomy, functioning, and pelvic health-related activities.

Throughout this book, we've examined the pelvic floor's complicated role in daily life, from core stability and bladder control to improved posture and sexual health. The importance of these exercises extends well beyond relieving symptoms; when performed on a regular basis, they provide the framework for a stronger, more robust body capable of moving smoothly and confidently through all stages of life.

You now have a collection of exercises, modifications, and practical strategies to help you achieve your specific objectives, such as recovery, pain management, or strength training. You have seen how Kegels, Bridge Pose, and other advanced routines may be tailored to your fitness level and lifestyle.

Remember that pelvic floor exercises do not always go in a straight line. Be patient with yourself, and celebrate little victories—each successful repetition, each moment of improved posture, and each feeling of enhanced control is a step forward. Consistency is key to getting long-term results, and even a few minutes each day may provide significant benefits over time.

If you have any questions or concerns as you continue on your journey, do not hesitate to seek help from competent professionals. Pelvic health physiotherapists and gynecologists may provide advise and changes to help you stay on track.

Finally, caring for your pelvic health means investing in your overall health, confidence, and quality of life. It is a personal commitment that becomes stronger with each practice. May this book be a foundation and companion in your journey to improved pelvic health, enabling you to live with more comfort, strength, and pleasure.

Thank you for dedicating this time to your health. Accept your journey with patience and care, understanding that you are building a stronger future one breath and exercise at a time.

Made in the USA
Columbia, SC
06 January 2025

51231707R00050